BBC good food eat well

VEGETARIAN
& VEGAN DISHES

10 9 8 7 6 5 4 3 2 1

BBC Books, an imprint of Ebury Publishing
20 Vauxhall Bridge Road,
London SW1V 2SA

BBC Books is part of the Penguin Random House group of companies whose addresses can be found at
global.penguinrandomhouse.com

Penguin
Random House
UK

Photographs © BBC Magazines 2017
Recipes © BBC Worldwide 2017
Book design © Woodlands Books Ltd 2017
All recipes contained in this book first appeared in BBC *Good Food* magazine.

First published by BBC Books in 2017

www.penguin.co.uk

A CIP catalogue record for this book is available from the British Library

ISBN 9781785941979

Printed and bound in China by Toppan Leefung

Project editor: Grace Paul
Design: Interstate Creative Partners Ltd and Kathryn Gammon
Cover Design: Interstate Creative Partners Ltd
Production: Alex Goddard
Picture Researcher: Gabby Harrington

Penguin Random House is committed to a sustainable
future for our business, our readers and our planet. This
book is made from Forest Stewardship Council® certified paper.

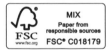

MIX
Paper from
responsible sources
FSC® C018179
www.fsc.org

PICTURE AND RECIPE CREDITS

BBC Books would like to thank the following people for providing photos. While every effort has been made to trace and
acknowledge all photographers, we should like to apologise should there be any errors or omissions.

Peter Cassidy p23, p31, p45, p47, p59, p67, p109, p165; Mike English p27, p61, p75, p79, p81, p83, p93, p101, p115, p121, p125,
p137, p139, p149, p191, p195, p201, p203, p209; Will Heap p37, p39, p95, p177, p205; Lara Holmes p131; Adrian Lawrence p183;
David Munns p55, p57, p63, p65, p85, p97, p135, p143, p147, p155, p163, p169; Myles New p77, p133, p141, p179; Stuart Ovenden
p33, p35, p113, p129, p145, p153, p157; Lis Parsons p69; Tom Regester p25, p41, p49, p103, p105, p111, p181; Toby Scott p127;
Roger Stowell p161, p175; Sam Stowell p51, p53, p87, p89, p91, p159, p173, p185, p189, p199, p207; Rob Streeter p13, p29, p43,
p73, p99, p117, p123, p151; Philip Webb p71, p171, p193; Clare Winfield p11, p15, p17, p19, p21, p187

All the recipes in this book were created by the editorial team at *Good Food* and by regular contributors to BBC Magazines.

good food eat well

VEGETARIAN & VEGAN DISHES

Editor **Miriam Nice**

BBC BOOKS

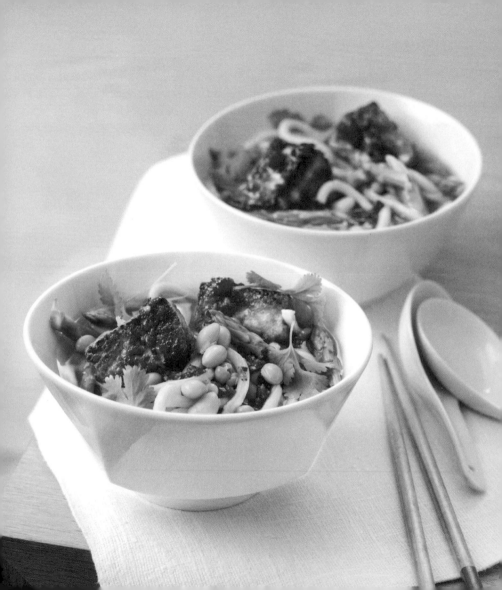

Contents

INTRODUCTION   6

Breakfast   10

Brunch & smoothies   34

Substantial soups & snacks   60

Lunch   100

Suppers   120

Healthy breads   160

Lighter bakes & puddings   170

INDEX   210

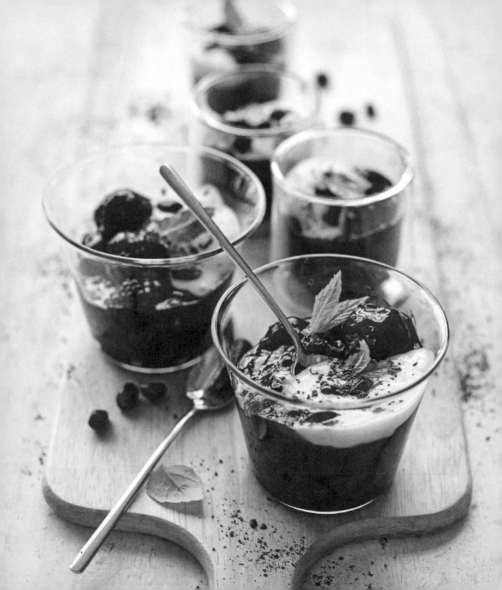

Introduction

. . . .

We get lots of requests for vegetarian and vegan recipes at *Good Food*. Whether the reasons for this are financial or just that some people want to eat less meat, we make sure we provide a balanced and ever-expanding range of recipe ideas for you.

If you're new to this type of cooking, we'll show you a few simple tricks that allow you to make rich sauces, gooey cakes and buttery biscuits. Without using animal products, for instance, creamy sauces can be made with coconut milk or nut butters. If you prefer to sweeten dishes without honey, try using maple syrup or agave nectar. Nutritional yeast mixed with ground almonds or cashews makes a miraculously 'cheesy' topping, that can be used in place of grated parmesan. Ingredients such as chia seeds and linseeds are good for binding biscuits and chewy cookies without using eggs.

Alongside these innovations you'll find some classic vegetarian and vegan-friendly dishes using veggie favourites like tofu and pulses. All recipes are vegetarian and wherever possible, we've adapted them or offered suggestions on how to make them vegan, too.

There are recipes here to cover groups of any size and occasion. Big batch cereals and smoothies to help you start the day right; quick meals, snacks and desserts for one alongside relaxed entertaining dishes for a crowd.

This is a book with heaps of inspiration for vegan and vegetarian cooking that everyone will want to try.

Miriam

Miriam Nice, Editor

Notes &
conversion tables

. . . .

NOTES ON THE RECIPES
- Eggs are large in the UK and Australia and extra large in America unless stated.
- Wash fresh produce before preparation.
- Recipes contain nutritional analyses for 'sugars', which means the total sugar content including all natural sugars in the ingredients, unless otherwise stated.

OVEN TEMPERATURES

GAS	°C	°C FAN	°F	OVEN TEMP.
¼	110	90	225	Very cool
½	120	100	250	Very cool
1	140	120	275	Cool or slow
2	150	130	300	Cool or slow
3	160	140	325	Warm
4	180	160	350	Moderate
5	190	170	375	Moderately hot
6	200	180	400	Fairly hot
7	220	200	425	Hot
8	230	210	450	Very hot
9	240	220	475	Very hot

APPROXIMATE WEIGHT CONVERSIONS
Cup measurements, which are used in Australia and America, have not been listed here as they vary from ingredient to ingredient. Kitchen scales should be used to measure dry/solid ingredients.

Good Food cares about sustainable sourcing and animal welfare. Where possible, humanely reared meats, sustainably caught fish (see fishonline.org for further information from the Marine Conservation Society) and free-range chickens and eggs are used when recipes are originally tested.

SPOON MEASURES

Spoon measurements are level unless otherwise specified.

- 1 teaspoon (tsp) = 5ml
- 1 tablespoon (tbsp) = 15ml
- 1 Australian tablespoon = 20ml (cooks in Australia should measure 3 teaspoons where 1 tablespoon is specified in a recipe)

APPROXIMATE LIQUID CONVERSIONS

METRIC	IMPERIAL	AUS	US
50ml	2fl oz	¼ cup	¼ cup
125ml	4fl oz	½ cup	½ cup
175ml	6fl oz	¾ cup	¾ cup
225ml	8fl oz	1 cup	1 cup
300ml	10fl oz/½ pint	½ pint	1¼ cups
450ml	16fl oz	2 cups	2 cups/1 pint
600ml	20fl oz/1 pint	1 pint	2½ cups
1 litre	35fl oz/1¾ pints	1¾ pints	1 quart

Cardamom & peach quinoa porridge

A satisfying, creamy porridge that's totally dairy-free.

PREP 3 mins COOK 20 mins 2

- 75g quinoa
- 25g porridge oats
- 4 cardamom pods
- 250ml unsweetened almond milk
- 2 ripe peaches, cut into slices
- 1 tsp maple syrup

1 Put the quinoa, oats and cardamom pods in a small saucepan with 250ml water and 100ml of the almond milk. Bring to the boil, then simmer gently for about 15 mins, stirring occasionally.

2 Pour in the remaining almond milk and cook for 5 mins more until creamy.

3 Remove the cardamom pods, spoon into bowls or jars, and top with the peaches and maple syrup.

GOOD TO KNOW: Vegan
PER SERVING kcal 231, fat 4g, saturates 1g, carbs 37g, sugars 10g, fibre 6g, protein 8g, salt 0.2g

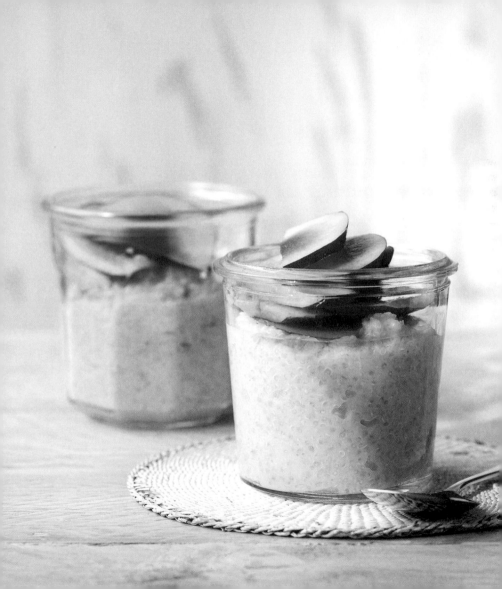

Rye bread with almond butter & pink grapefruit segments

A quick and balanced breakfast, perfect for busy mornings.

PREP 3 mins COOK 3 mins 2

- 1 grapefruit (you will need about 100g flesh)
- 4 tbsp almond butter
- 2 slices rye bread, toasted or untoasted

1 Segment the grapefruit and spoon the fruit, along with any juice, into a small bowl.
2 Spread the almond butter onto the rye bread, and top with the grapefruit, drizzling any juice over the top.

GOOD TO KNOW: Vegan
PER SERVING kcal 333, fat 18g, saturates 2g, carbs 30g, sugars 7g, fibre 8g, protein 10g, salt 0.8g

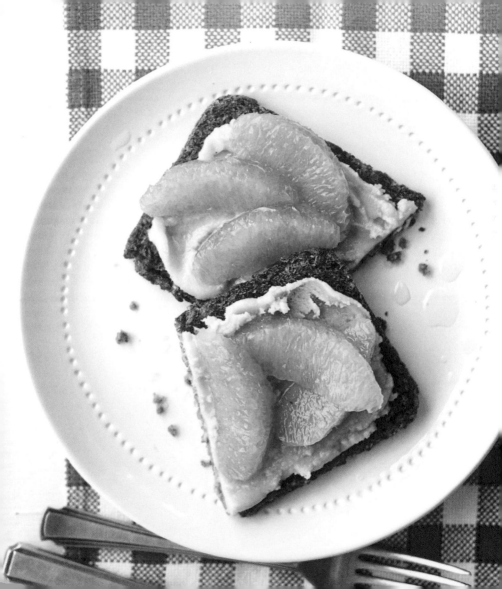

Nutty cinnamon & apple granola

Get ahead and create your own big batch of crunchy toasted granola with a hint of spice. It will keep for a month in an airtight jar.

PREP 10 mins COOK 20 mins   12

- 400g jumbo oats
- 2 tsp ground cinnamon
- 150g dried apple, roughly chopped
- 150g coconut oil, melted
- 250g pack mixed nuts, roughly chopped
- 100ml maple syrup

1 Heat oven to 180C/160C fan/gas 4. Line 2 large baking trays with baking parchment. Mix all the ingredients together except the maple syrup. Spread the granola out on the trays and drizzle over the maple syrup.

2 Bake in the oven for 20 mins, stirring the granola well halfway through so that it cooks evenly. Leave to cool before storing in a jar or airtight container. Best eaten within 1 month.

GOOD TO KNOW: *Vegan*
PER SERVING kcal 407, fat 26g, saturates 12g, carbs 34g, sugars 12g, fibre 5g, protein 8g, salt 0g

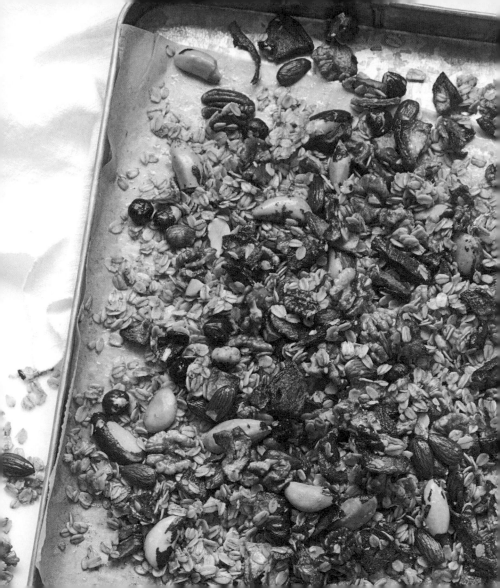

Cranberry & almond clusters

This nutty batch of gluten-free cereal is great served with soya or coconut yogurt.

PREP 5 mins COOK 5 mins 10

- 50g honey
- 200g flaked almonds
- 225g pack puffed brown rice (we used Rude Health)
- 200g cranberries

1 Heat the honey in a frying pan until it loosens and starts to bubble, then stir in the flaked almonds. Cook for a few mins, stirring constantly, so that some of the almonds toast and turn golden.

2 Tip the almonds onto baking parchment, leave to cool, then break into clusters. Mix with the puffed rice and cranberries, then store in a jar or airtight container. Best eaten within 3 weeks.

GOOD TO KNOW: Vegetarian
PER SERVING kcal 230, fat 12g, saturates 1g, carbs 24g, sugars 5g, fibre 2g, protein 7g, salt 0g

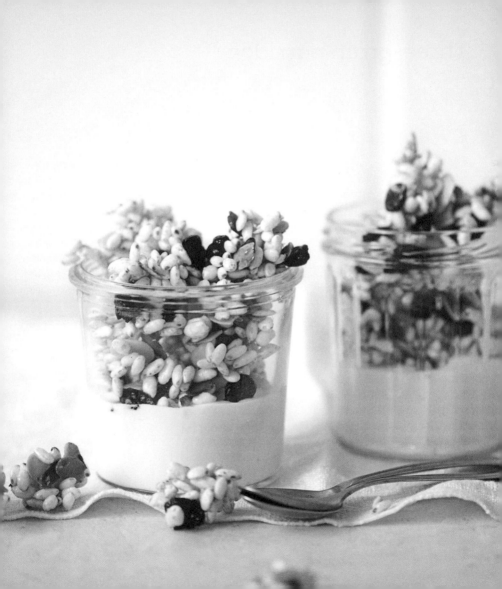

Three-grain porridge

Toasting the grains is well worth the effort for maximum flavour.

🕐 PREP 5 mins COOK 10 mins 🕐 18

- 300g oatmeal
- 300g spelt flakes
- 300g barley flakes
- agave nectar and sliced strawberries, to serve (optional)

1 Working in batches, toast the oatmeal, spelt flakes and barley in a large, dry frying pan for 5 mins until golden, then leave to cool and store in an airtight container.

2 When you want to eat it, simply combine 50g of the porridge mixture in a saucepan with 300ml almond milk or water. Cook for 5 mins, stirring occasionally, then top with a drizzle of agave nectar and strawberries, if you like. Will keep for 6 months.

GOOD TO KNOW: Vegan
PER SERVING kcal 179, fat 2g, saturates 0g, carbs 32g, sugars 1g, fibre 4g, protein 7g, salt 0g

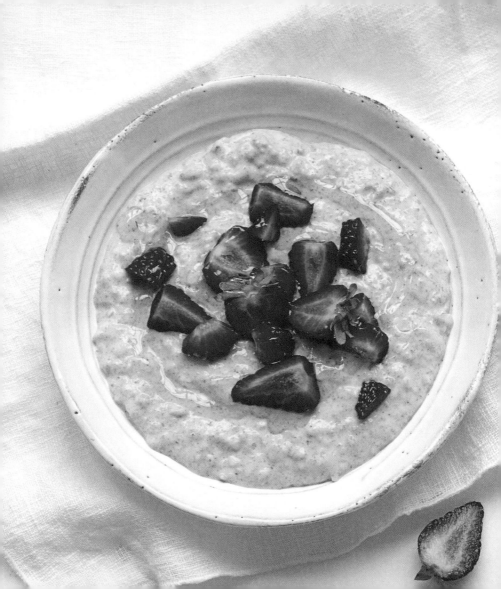

Homemade cocoa pops

A crunchy, chocolatey cereal everyone will love.

🕐 PREP 10 mins COOK 15 mins 🥧 20

- 100g coconut oil
- 200g honey
- 100g cocoa powder
- 850g buckwheat
- 150g pack cacao nibs (you can substitute with chopped dark chocolate)

1 Heat oven to 180C/160C fan/gas 4. Line 2 large baking trays with baking parchment. In a large microwaveable bowl, melt the coconut oil with the honey, cocoa powder and a pinch of sea salt.
2 Stir in the buckwheat, covering well in the chocolate mixture.
3 Spread the mixture onto the baking trays and bake for 15 mins, stirring halfway, then mix in the cacao nibs. Allow to cool before storing in a Kilner jar or airtight container. Best eaten within 1 month.

GOOD TO KNOW: Vegetarian
PER SERVING kcal 302, fat 11g, saturates 7g, carbs 44g, sugars 8g, fibre 4g, protein 6g, salt 0g

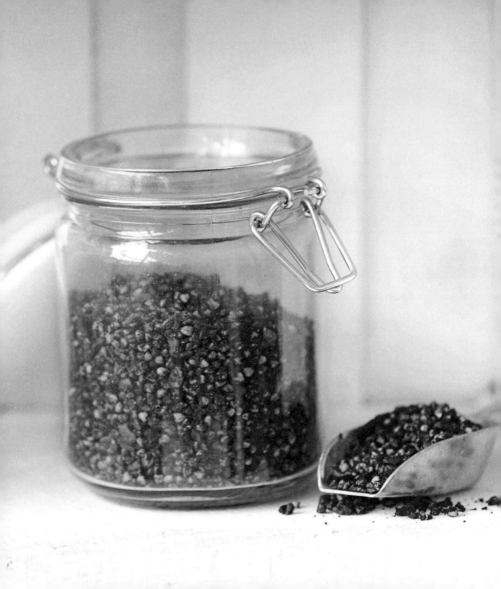

Raspberry ripple chia pudding

A creamy alternative to porridge, perfect for hot summer mornings.

🕐 PREP 15 mins   🍽 2

- 50g white chia seeds
- 200ml coconut drinking milk
- 1 nectarine or peach, cut into slices
- 2 tbsp goji berries

FOR THE RASPBERRY PURÉE

- 100g raspberries
- 1 tsp lemon juice
- 2 tsp maple syrup

1 Divide the chia seeds and coconut milk between 2 serving bowls and stir well. Leave to soak for 5 mins, stirring occasionally, until the seeds swell and thicken when stirred.

2 Meanwhile, combine the purée ingredients in a small food processor, or blitz with a hand blender. Swirl a spoonful into each bowl, then arrange the nectarine or peach slices on top and scatter with the goji berries.

GOOD TO KNOW: Vegan
PER SERVING kcal 257, fat 10g, saturates 3g, carbs 26g, sugars 22g, fibre 13g, protein 8g, salt 0.2g

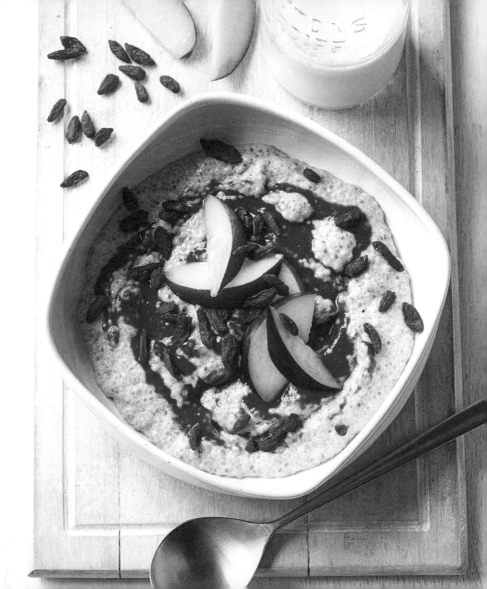

Matcha breakfast bowl

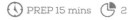

This vibrant green-tea yogurt is packed with fresh fruit. Use dairy-free yogurt to make it vegan.

🕐 PREP 15 mins 🥧 2

- 300g natural yogurt
- 1 tbsp matcha powder
- 2 tsp maple syrup
- 1 kiwi fruit, sliced
- 1 peach, sliced
- 100g blueberries
- 20g coconut flakes, toasted

Mix the yogurt with the matcha and maple syrup, and divide between 2 bowls. Top with the kiwi, peach and blueberries. Sprinkle over the coconut flakes just before serving.

GOOD TO KNOW: Vegetarian
PER SERVING kcal 261, fat 11g, saturates 8g, carbs 27g, sugars 26g, fibre 5g, protein 10g, salt 0.3g

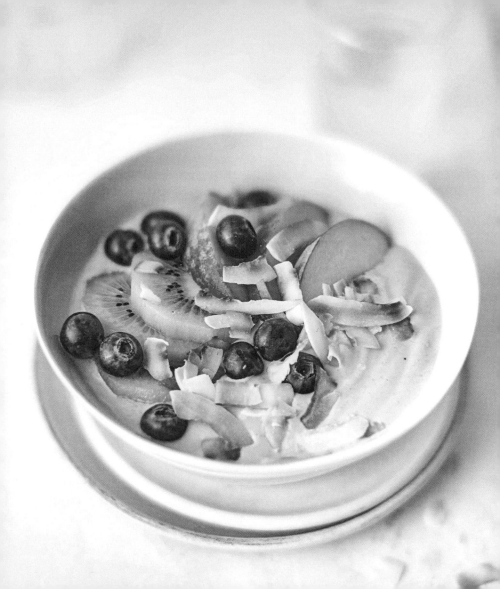

Orange & blueberry Bircher

A delicious breakfast that's ready when you get up? What's not to like!

🕐 PREP 5 mins plus overnight chillling 🍽 2

- 70g porridge oats
- 2 tbsp golden linseeds
- zest of ½ orange
- 175g pot yogurt
- 2 peeled and chopped oranges
- 4 handfuls blueberries

Mix the oats and golden linseeds with the orange zest. Pour over 300ml boiling water and leave overnight. The next day, stir in three-quarters of the yogurt, spoon into glasses or bowls, top with the orange pieces, the remaining yogurt and blueberries.

GOOD TO KNOW: Vegetarian
PER SERVING kcal 345, fat 9g, saturates 3g, carbs 48g, sugars 22g, fibre 8g, protein 13g, salt 0.2g

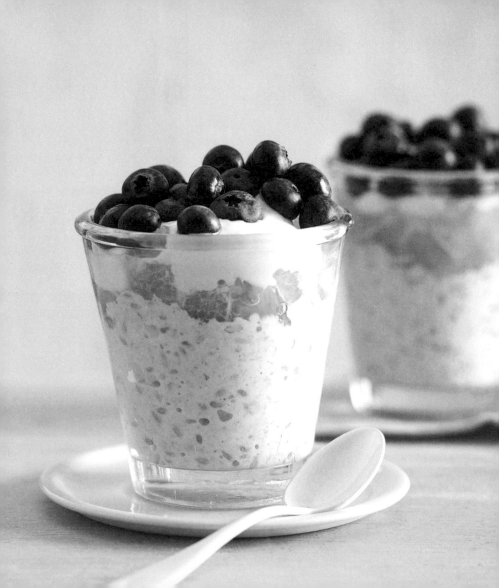

Breakfast muffins

A healthier version of a classic blueberry muffin – perfect for busy days.

PREP 15 mins COOK 30 mins   MAKES 12

- 2 large eggs
- 150g pot natural low-fat yogurt
- 50ml extra virgin rapeseed oil
- 100g apple sauce or puréed apples (in the baby food aisle)
- 1 ripe banana, mashed
- 4 tbsp clear honey
- 1 tsp vanilla extract
- 200g wholemeal flour
- 50g rolled oats, plus extra for sprinkling
- 1½ tsp baking powder
- 1½ tsp bicarbonate of soda
- 1½ tsp cinnamon
- 100g blueberries
- 2 tbsp mixed seeds (we used pumpkin, sunflower and flaxseed)

1 Heat oven to 180C/160C fan/gas 4. Line a 12-hole muffin tin with 12 large muffin cases. In a jug, mix the eggs, yogurt, oil, apple sauce, banana, honey and vanilla. Tip the remaining ingredients, except the seeds, into a large bowl, add a pinch of salt and mix to combine.

2 Pour the wet ingredients into the dry and mix briefly until you have a smooth batter – don't overmix as this will make the muffins heavy. Divide the batter among the cases. Sprinkle the muffins with the extra oats and the seeds. Bake for 25–30 mins until golden and well risen, and a skewer inserted into the centre of a muffin comes out clean. Remove from the oven, transfer to a wire rack and leave to cool. Can be stored in a sealed container for up to 3 days.

GOOD TO KNOW: Vegetarian
PER SERVING kcal 179, fat 7g, saturates 1g, carbs 23g, sugars 10g, fibre 3g, protein 5g, salt 0.6g

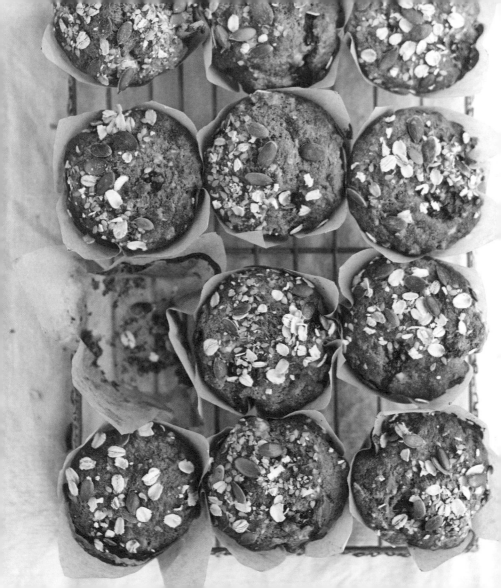

Clementine & honey couscous

· ·

Use frozen raspberries when fresh ones are out of season. For a vegan version, go for dairy-free alternatives to the yogurt and butter and maple syrup in place of honey.

🕐 PREP 20 mins COOK 10 mins 🍽 4

- 100g pistachio or other nuts
- 300g couscous
- ¼ tsp ground cinnamon, plus more to serve
- 8 clementines (seedless are best)
- 1 tsp butter
- 2 tbsp runny honey, plus more to serve
- 1 tsp orange flower water (optional)
- 300g fresh or frozen raspberries
- 500g pot reduced-fat Greek-style yogurt, to serve

1 Heat the oven to 200C/180C fan/gas 6. Spread the nuts over a baking sheet and toast for 5-8 mins until pale golden. Meanwhile, put the couscous and cinnamon into a large bowl. Finely grate the zest from 2 clementines, then squeeze their juice into a pan with the zest. Add the butter, honey and 200ml water and bring to the boil. Pour this over the couscous, cover with cling film, then leave to absorb for 10 mins.

2 Using a serrated knife, peel, then thinly slice the remaining clementines. Sprinkle with the orange flower water, if using. Roughly chop the nuts.

3 Fluff up the couscous with a fork, then mix in most of the nuts.

4 Serve the couscous in bowls, topped with the clementines and raspberries. Eat with a spoonful of yogurt, an extra sprinkle of cinnamon and nuts and a squeeze of honey.

· ·
GOOD TO KNOW: Vegetarian
PER SERVING kcal 333, fat 9g, saturates 2g, carbs 50g, sugars 16g, fibre 8g, protein 11g, salt 0.1g

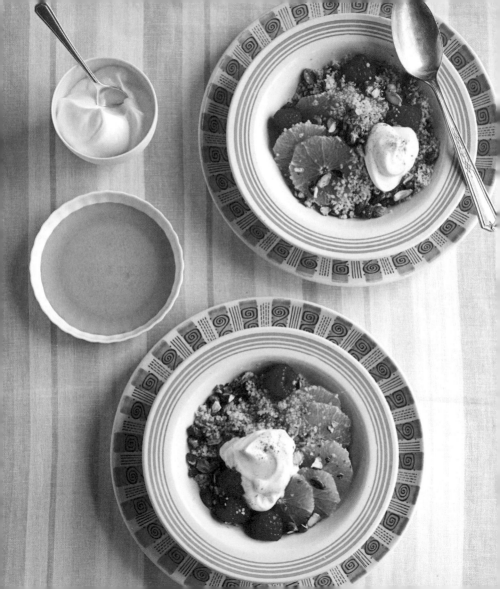

Summer fruit compote

· ·

A nutritious fruity breakfast mix, delicious on its own, or stirred through your favourite yogurt or porridge.

🕐 PREP 5 mins COOK 10 mins 🥧 4

- 4 large plums, stoned and cut into wedges
- 200g punnet blueberries
- zest and juice 1 orange
- 25g soft light brown sugar
- 150g punnet raspberries
- thick yogurt and honey or maple syrup, to serve (optional)

1 Cook the plums and blueberries in a small pan with the orange zest and juice, sugar and 4 tbsp water until slightly softened but not mushy. Gently stir in the raspberries and cook for 1 min more.

2 Remove from the heat and allow to cool to room temperature. Serve with yogurt and a drizzle of honey or syrup, if you like.

· ·
GOOD TO KNOW: Vegan (without yogurt or honey)
PER SERVING kcal 98, fat 0g, saturates 0g, carbs 22g, sugars 21g, fibre 4g, protein 2g, salt 0g

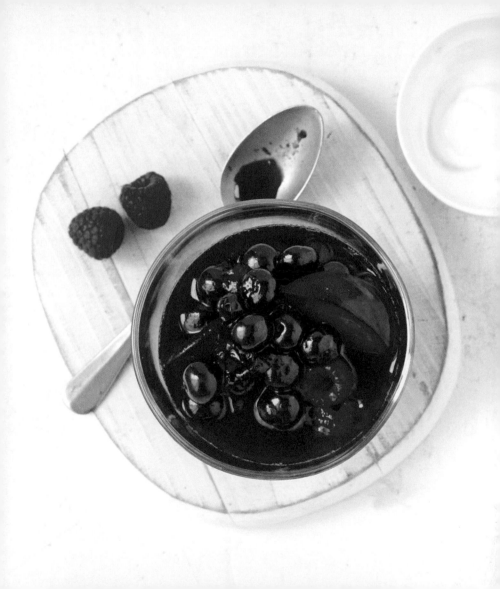

Immune boosting smoothie

Baobab adds a tangy flavour, antioxidants and vitamin C, but this smoothie is still delicious without it. Use agave nectar instead of honey if you prefer.

🕐 PREP 5 mins 🕐 1

- 100g coconut yogurt
- 3 tbsp unsweetened almond milk
- ½ tsp ground turmeric
- 3cm piece of fresh ginger, peeled
- 2 tsp baobab powder (optional, find it in health food shops)
- 1 small ripe banana
- 1 tsp honey
- 1 tbsp oats
- juice of ½ lemon

Put the coconut yogurt and almond milk into a high-speed blender, then add the turmeric, fresh ginger and baobab powder (if using). Tip in the remaining ingredients, then blend again until smooth. Add a handful of ice and blitz if you prefer a colder drink. Pour into glasses to serve.

GOOD TO KNOW: *Vegetarian*
PER SERVING kcal 359, fat 19g, saturates 13g, carbs 38g, sugars 24g, fibre 3g, protein 6g, salt 0.1g

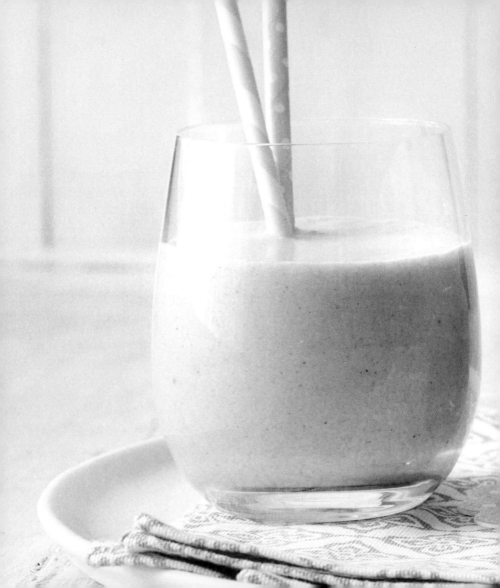

Clean green smoothie

A natural energy boost for mornings that need a bit more of a kick-start.

🕐 PREP 5 mins 🍽 1

- 250ml unsweetened almond milk
- 1 tbsp ground flaxseed
- 1 tsp maca powder (optional)
- pinch ground cinnamon
- 1 Medjool date, stoned
- 1 small ripe banana
- handful cavolo nero or spinach
- 1 tbsp almond butter

Pour the almond milk into a high-speed blender then add the ground flaxseed, maca powder (if using) and the cinnamon. Add the remaining ingredients then blitz until smooth. Pour into glasses and serve.

GOOD TO KNOW: Vegan
PER SERVING kcal 329, fat 15g, saturates 1g, carbs 36g, sugars 33g, fibre 8g, protein 8g, salt 0.4g

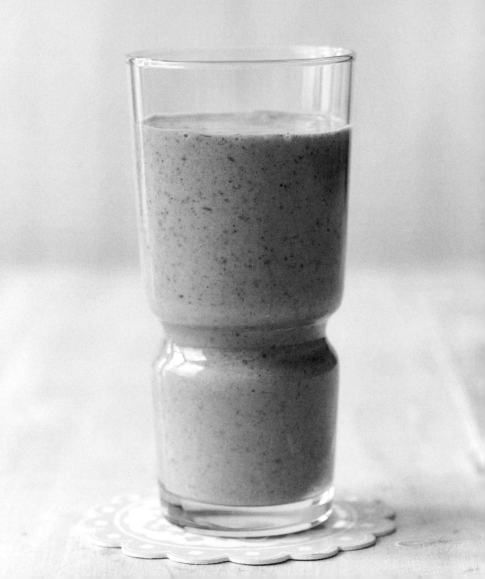

Winter warmer smoothie

Fresh ginger gives this beetroot and blackberry smoothie a spicy kick – perfect for an early morning or afternoon pick-me-up.

🕐 PREP 5 mins   🥤 1

- 250ml coconut water
- pinch ground cinnamon
- ¼ tsp ground nutmeg
- 4cm piece fresh ginger, peeled
- 1 tbsp shelled hemp seeds
- 2 small cooked beetroot, roughly chopped
- small handful blackberries
- 1 pear, roughly chopped
- small handful kale

Pour the coconut water into your blender with the spices and fresh ginger. Tip in the remaining ingredients and blend until smooth. Add more liquid if you prefer a thinner consistency. Pour into glasses and serve.

GOOD TO KNOW: Vegan
PER SERVING kcal 238, fat 6g, saturates 1g, carbs 37g, sugars 34g, fibre 8g, protein 5g, salt 0.3g

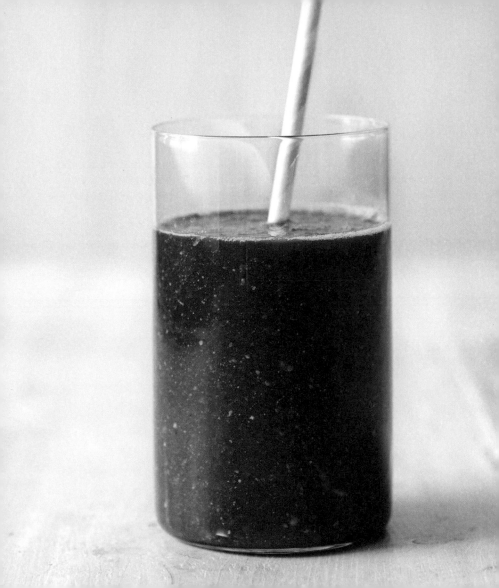

Sunshine smoothie

A ray of sun in a glass, and it provides two of your five-a-day, too!

🕐 PREP 5 mins   🍶 3

- 500ml carrot juice, chilled
- 200g pineapple (fresh or canned)
- 2 bananas, broken into chunks
- small piece ginger, peeled
- 20g cashew nuts
- juice 1 lime

Put the ingredients in a blender and whizz until smooth. Drink straight away or pour into a bottle to drink on the go. Will keep in the fridge for a day.

GOOD TO KNOW: Vegan
PER SERVING kcal 171, fat 4g, saturates 1g, carbs 30g, sugars 27g, fibre 3g, protein 3g, salt 0.2g

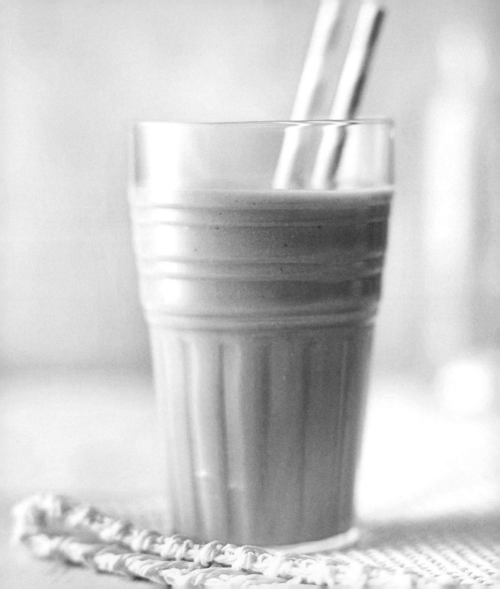

Minty pineapple smoothie

For an even creamier blend soak the cashews overnight in water, drain and rinse the next day.

🕐 PREP 10 mins   🍴 2

- 200g pineapple, peeled, cored and cut into chunks
- a few mint leaves
- 50g baby spinach leaves
- 25g oats
- 2 tbsp linseeds
- handful unsalted, unroasted cashew nuts
- fresh lime juice, to taste

Put all the ingredients in a blender with 200ml water and blend until smooth. If it's too thick, add more water (up to 400ml) until you get the right mix.

GOOD TO KNOW: Vegan
PER SERVING kcal 177, fat 8g, saturates 1g, carbs 19g, sugars 11g, fibre 4g, protein 6g, salt 0.1g

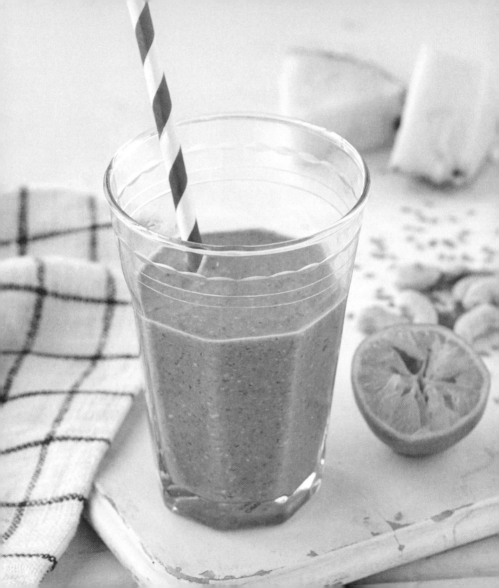

Tropical smoothie bowl

A bowl of fruit heaven, suitable for vegans.

PREP 20 mins 2

- 1 small ripe mango, stoned, peeled and cut into chunks
- 200g pineapple, peeled, cored and cut into chunks
- 2 ripe bananas
- 2 tbsp coconut yogurt (not coconut-flavoured yogurt)
- 150ml coconut drinking milk
- 2 passion fruits, halved, seeds scooped out
- handful blueberries
- 2 tbsp coconut flakes
- a few mint leaves

Put the mango, pineapple, bananas, yogurt and coconut milk in a blender, and blitz until smooth and thick. Pour into 2 bowls and decorate with the passion fruit, blueberries, coconut flakes and mint leaves. Will keep in the fridge for 1 day. Add the toppings just before serving.

GOOD TO KNOW: Vegan
PER SERVING kcal 332, fat 15g, saturates 13g, carbs 41g, sugars 38g, fibre 8g, protein 4g, salt 0.1g

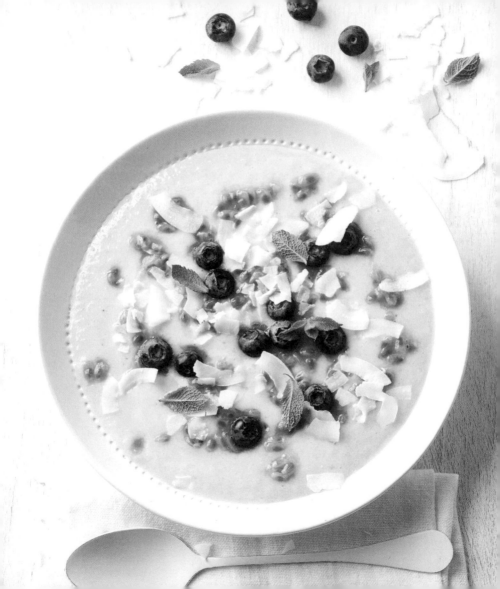

Green rainbow smoothie bowl

Choose a ripe avocado to make this smoothie bowl perfectly rich and creamy.

🕐 PREP 20 mins 🍽 2

- 50g spinach
- 1 avocado, stoned, peeled and halved
- 1 ripe mango, stoned, peeled and cut into chunks
- 1 apple, cored and cut into chunks
- 200ml almond milk
- 1 dragon fruit, peeled and cut into even chunks
- 100g mixed berries (we used strawberries, raspberries and blueberries)

Put the spinach, avocado, mango, apple and almond milk in a blender, and blitz until smooth and thick. Divide between 2 bowls and top with the dragon fruit and berries.

GOOD TO KNOW: Vegan
PER SERVING kcal 251, fat 16g, saturates 3g, carbs 19g, sugars 18g, fibre 7g, protein 4g, salt 0.2g

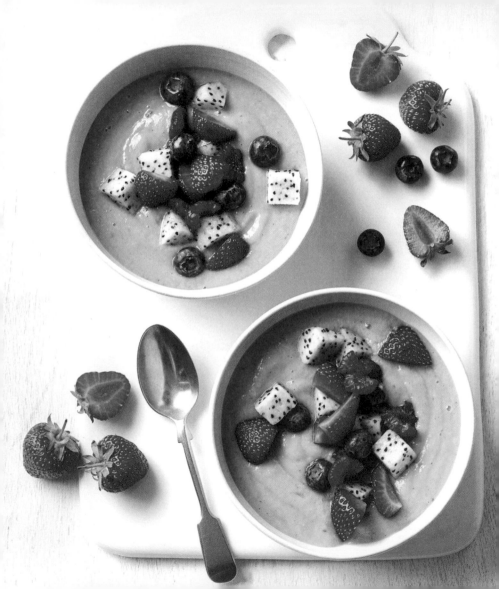

Protein pancake stack

· ·

The perfect fuel after exercise or great for a weekend treat.

🕐 PREP 20 mins COOK 20 mins 🥧 2

FOR THE BATTER
- 2 tbsp ground flaxseeds
- 20g ground almonds
- 300ml soya milk
- 200g quinoa flour
- 1 medium banana, mashed
- 2 tbsp maple syrup
- coconut oil, for frying

FOR THE BLUEBERRY CHIA JAM (MAKES 200ML)
- 200g blueberries, mashed
- 2 tbsp chia seeds
- 1-2 tbsp maple syrup, to taste
- 2 tsp lemon juice

FOR THE STACK
- 100g coconut yogurt or Greek yogurt
- mixed berries
- 1 tbsp pistachio nuts or pumpkin seeds, chopped, toasted if you like
- 2 tsp hulled hemp seeds

1 In a bowl stir the flaxseeds with 6 tbsp water and leave to soak. Meanwhile, make the jam. In a pan over a medium heat, mash the blueberries with a fork and heat until bubbling. Off the heat, stir in the chia seeds, maple syrup and lemon juice, then leave to cool.

2 Put the ground almonds, milk, flour, banana, maple syrup, a pinch of salt and the flaxseed mixture in a blender and blitz until smooth.

3 Fry the pancakes in a large frying pan in batches, using 1 tsp coconut oil for each batch. Flip over when the edges are browning and bubbles have formed on top, then cook for another few mins until golden. Keep warm while you cook the rest of the batches.

4 Layer the pancakes with the blueberry jam, yogurt and mixed berries, then scatter with nuts and seeds.

· ·
GOOD TO KNOW: Vegan
PER SERVING kcal 798, fat 32g, saturates 8g, carbs 91g, sugars 39g, fibre 15g, protein 29g, salt 0.3g

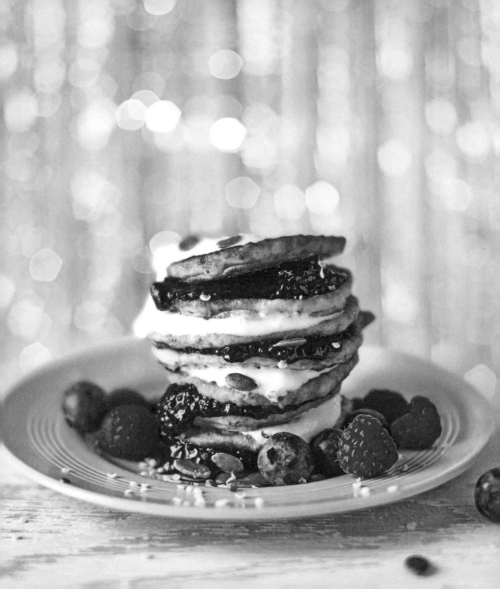

Manakeesh

Packed with Middle Eastern flavours, this dish makes a quick brunch or light lunch. Use coconut yogurt and marinated tofu instead of feta to make this dairy-free.

PREP 30 mins COOK 10 mins | 4

- 4 lavash or wholemeal flatbreads
- 200g pack feta

FOR THE SALAD
- 1 tomato, chopped
- ½ cucumber, chopped
- ½ small pack mint, leaves only
- 15 pitted black olives
- balsamic vinegar, for drizzling
- extra virgin olive oil, for drizzling

FOR THE GARLIC YOGURT
- 1 garlic clove, crushed
- 150ml pot natural yogurt

FOR THE DRESSING
- ½ bunch oregano, chopped
- bunch thyme, leaves only
- 150ml olive oil
- 1 garlic clove, crushed
- juice ½ lemon
- ¼ tsp sumac
- 1 tsp sesame seeds, toasted

1 First, make the salad. Put the tomato, cucumber, mint and olives in a large bowl, drizzle over a little balsamic vinegar and some extra virgin olive oil, then mix to combine. Season to taste.

2 Stir the crushed garlic into the yogurt and mix thoroughly, then season and set aside.

3 To make the dressing, put the oregano, thyme, olive oil and garlic in a jug and blend with a stick blender. Add the lemon juice, sumac, sesame seeds and some seasoning, and stir well. Spread one side of each flatbread with 2 heaped tbsp of the dressing, then top each with a quarter of the feta.

4 Fold the flatbreads in half or roll up and lightly fry each on both sides in a dry griddle pan over a medium heat until lightly toasted and golden. Keep warm on a low heat in the oven while you fry the others. Serve with a pile of the salad and garnish with a dollop of the garlic yogurt.

GOOD TO KNOW: Vegetarian
PER SERVING kcal 761, fat 54g, saturates 14g, carbs 47g, sugars 9g, fibre 5g, protein 20g, salt 2.6g

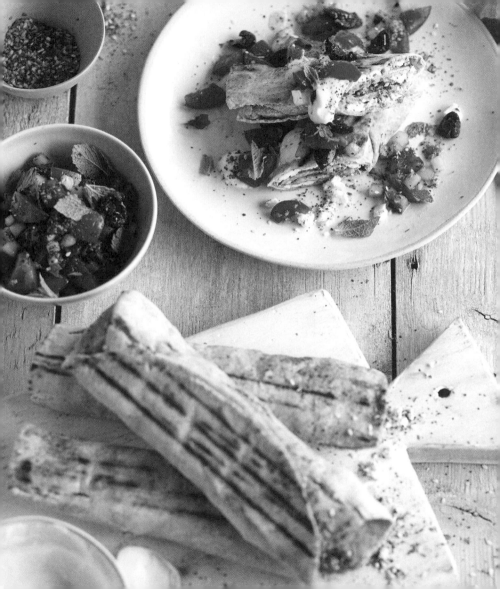

Smoky beans on toast

This filling brunch dish packs in four of your five-a-day.

🕐 PREP 5 mins COOK 30 mins 🥧 1

- ½ tbsp olive oil, plus extra for drizzling
- ½ small onion, sliced
- ½ small red pepper, thinly sliced into strips
- 1 garlic clove, halved
- 227g can chopped tomatoes
- ½ tsp smoked paprika
- 2 tsp red wine vinegar
- 210g can butter beans or chickpeas, drained
- ¼ tsp sugar
- 1 slice seeded bread
- a few parsley sprigs, finely chopped

1 Heat the oil in a small pan, add the onion and pepper, and fry gently until soft, about 10-15 mins. Crush half the garlic and add this to the pan, along with the tomatoes, paprika, vinegar, beans, sugar and some seasoning. Bring to a simmer and cook for 10-15 mins or until slightly reduced and thickened.

2 Toast the bread, rub with the remaining garlic and drizzle with a little oil. Spoon the beans over the toast, drizzle with a little more oil and scatter over the parsley.

GOOD TO KNOW: Vegan
PER SERVING kcal 460, fat 19g, saturates 3g, carbs 49g, sugars 17g, fibre 14g, protein 15g, salt 1.1g

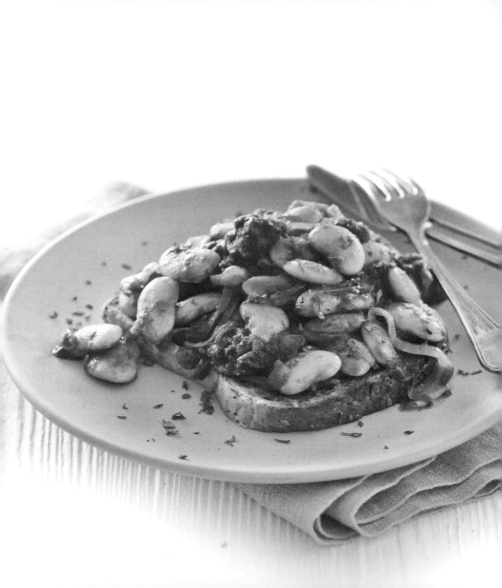

Tofu brekkie pancakes

Silken tofu magically helps create these thick American-style pancakes without eggs or dairy.

PREP 10 mins COOK 10 mins 4-6

- 50g Brazil nuts, toasted and chopped
- sliced banana, to serve
- berries, to serve
- maple syrup, to serve

FOR THE BATTER
- 349g pack firm silken tofu
- 2 tsp vanilla extract
- 2 tsp lemon juice
- 400ml unsweetened almond milk
- 1 tbsp vegetable oil, plus 1-2 tbsp extra for frying
- 250g buckwheat flour
- 4 tbsp light muscovado sugar
- 1½ tsp ground mixed spice
- 1 tbsp gluten-free baking powder

1 Put the tofu, vanilla, lemon juice and 200ml of the milk into a jug or bowl. Using a stick blender, blend until thick like yogurt. Stir in the oil and the rest of the milk to loosen. Put the dry ingredients and 1 tsp salt in a bowl and whisk together. Make a well in the centre and stir in the tofu mixture.

2 Heat 1 tsp oil in a non-stick frying pan. Ladle in the batter to make pancakes that are about 12cm across. Cook for 2 mins or until bubbles pop up over the surface. Flip over the pancakes and cook for 1 min more or until puffed up.

3 Keep the panckes warm while you cook the remaining batter, using a little more oil each time. Serve with the toasted nuts, sliced banana, berries and a little maple syrup.

GOOD TO KNOW: Vegan
PER SERVING kcal 343, fat 14g, saturates 2g, carbs 41g, sugars 15g, fibre 5g, protein 11g, salt 1.6g

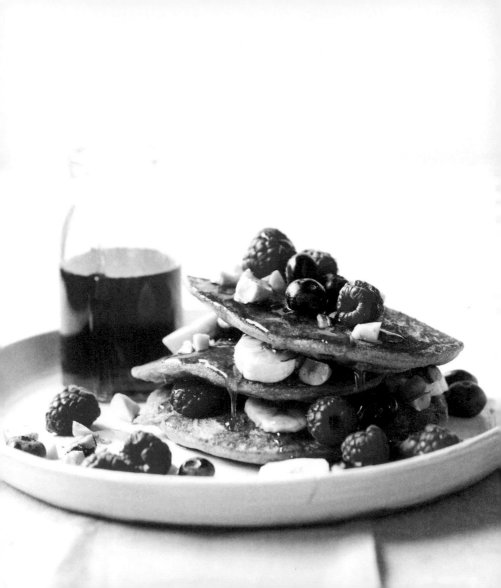

Vegan tomato & mushroom pancakes

Delicate pancakes with a creamy tomato and button mushroom topping.

🕐 PREP 5 mins COOK 30 mins 🍽 2

- 140g white self-raising flour
- 1 tsp soya flour
- 400ml soya milk
- vegetable oil, for frying

FOR THE TOPPING
- 2 tbsp vegetable oil
- 250g button mushrooms
- 250g cherry tomatoes, halved
- 2 tbsp soya cream or soya milk
- large handful pine nuts
- snipped chives, to serve

1 Sift the flours and a pinch of salt into a blender. Add the soya milk and blend to make a smooth batter.

2 Heat a little oil in a medium non-stick frying pan until very hot. Pour about 3 tbsp of the batter into the pan and cook over a medium heat until bubbles appear on the surface of the pancake. Flip the pancake over with a palette knife and cook the other side until golden brown. Repeat with the remaining batter, keeping the cooked pancakes warm as you go. You will make about 8.

3 For the topping, heat the oil in a frying pan. Cook the mushrooms until tender, add the tomatoes and cook for a couple of mins. Pour in the soya cream or milk and pine nuts, then gently cook until combined. Divide the pancakes between 2 plates, then spoon over the tomatoes and mushrooms and scatter with chives.

GOOD TO KNOW: Vegan
PER SERVING kcal 609, fat 35g, saturates 4g, carbs 59g, sugars 6g, fibre 6g, protein 18g, salt 0.87g

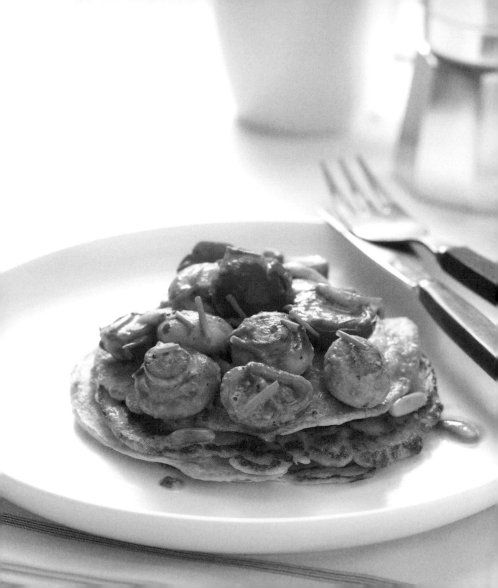

Sweetcorn beignets

Feeding a crowd? Just add a bowl of sliced avocado, some grilled ripe tomatoes and a pot of coffee for a fantastic help-yourself brunch.

🕐 PREP 10 mins COOK 25 mins   🥧 MAKES 20

- 3 sweetcorn cobs, cooked, kernels sliced off
- 200g tapioca flour
- 150g polenta
- ½ tsp bicarbonate of soda
- ¼ tsp garlic powder
- ¼ tsp chilli flakes
- 1 tsp cumin seeds, toasted
- 330ml cider
- sunflower oil, for frying
- flaky sea salt, to serve

FOR THE SALSA

- 1 tbsp extra virgin rapeseed oil
- 2 medium courgettes, finely diced
- 1 green chilli, diced
- 1 garlic clove, grated
- 1 green tomato, diced
- 1 tsp chopped coriander
- juice 1 lime

1 For the salsa, heat the oil in a frying pan over a medium heat and fry the courgette for 3 mins or until lightly coloured. Off the heat mix in the chilli, garlic, tomato and coriander. Leave to cool, then add the lime juice and season to taste.

2 Whizz a third of the corn kernels in a food processor until smooth, then tip into a large bowl with the tapioca, polenta, bicarb, garlic, spices and seasoning. Whisk in the cider and remaining sweetcorn.

3 Heat a deep-fat fryer (or oil in a large saucepan) to 180C. Working in batches, deep-fry spoonfuls of the batter for 1-2 mins or until golden, then lift out with a slotted spoon onto a baking tray lined with kitchen paper. Sprinkle with salt and serve with the salsa. Visit bbcgoodfood.com for a guide to deep-frying safely.

GOOD TO KNOW: Vegetarian
PER SERVING kcal 124, fat 6g, saturates 1g, carbs 13g, sugars 2g, fibre 2g, protein 2g, salt 0.2g

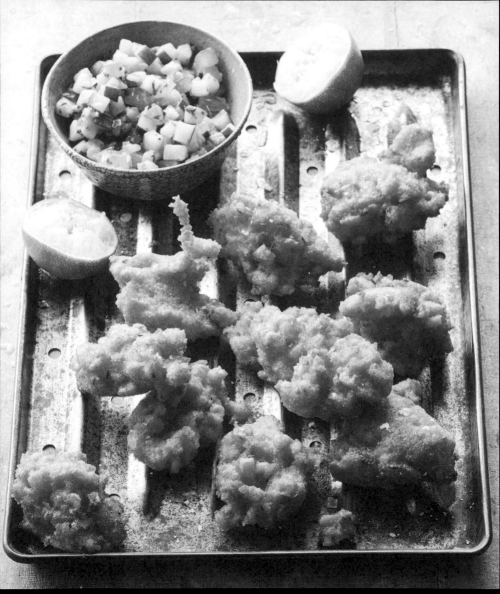

Summer carrot, tarragon & white bean soup

· ·

This satisfying summer soup is freezable so you can enjoy a quick and easy lunch another day.

🕐 PREP 10 mins COOK 20 mins 🥧 4

- 1 tbsp extra virgin rapeseed oil
- 2 large leeks, well washed, halved lengthways and finely sliced
- 700g carrots, chopped
- 1.4 litres hot reduced-salt vegetable bouillon (we used Marigold)
- 4 garlic cloves, finely grated
- 2 x 400g cans cannellini beans in water
- 2/3 small pack tarragon, leaves roughly chopped

1 Heat the oil over a medium heat in a large pan and fry the leeks and carrots for 5 mins to soften.
2 Pour over the stock, stir in the garlic, the beans with their liquid, and three-quarters of the tarragon, then cover and simmer for 15 mins or until the veg is just tender. Stir in the remaining tarragon before serving.

· ·

GOOD TO KNOW: Vegan
PER SERVING kcal 271, fat 6g, saturates 1g, carbs 38g, sugars 17g, fibre 13g, protein 11g, salt 0.7g

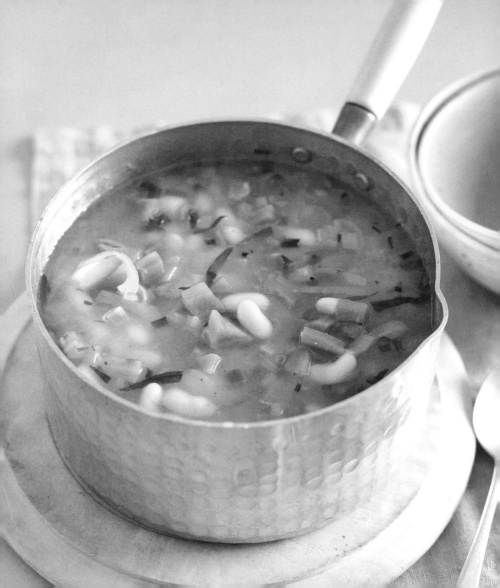

Spicy harissa, aubergine & chickpea soup

. . . .

Healthy, hot and peppery.

🕐 PREP 10 mins COOK 40 mins 🍴 4

- 1 onion, chopped
- 1 tbsp olive oil
- 2 tbsp harissa
- 2 aubergines, diced
- 400g can chopped tomatoes
- 400g can chickpeas, drained
- 2 tbsp coriander, chopped

Soften the onion in olive oil in a large saucepan, then add the harissa and cook for 2 mins, stirring. Add the aubergines and coat in the harissa. Add the tomatoes, chickpeas and 500ml of water. Bring to the boil and simmer for 30 mins. Stir through the coriander, season and serve.

GOOD TO KNOW: Vegan
PER SERVING kcal 157, fat 5g, saturates 1g, carbs 20g, sugars 8g, fibre 9g, protein 6g, salt 0.7g

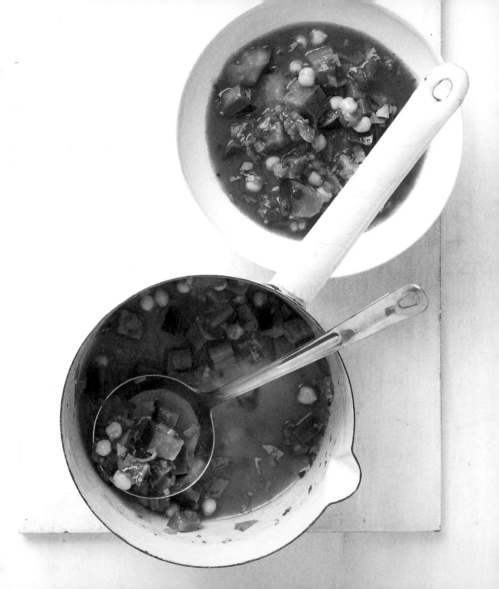

Butternut soup with crispy sage & apple croutons

· ·

An autumnal starter everyone can enjoy. Some sherry is vegan, but check before buying or replace with extra vegetable stock.

PREP 20 mins COOK 40 mins 4

- 1 tbsp olive oil
- 1 large onion, chopped
- 1 garlic clove, chopped
- 1 butternut squash, about 1kg, peeled, deseeded and chopped
- 3 tbsp madeira or dry sherry
- 500ml gluten-free vegetable stock, plus a little extra if necessary
- 1 tsp chopped sage, plus 20 small leaves, cleaned and dried
- sunflower oil, for frying
- 1 apple, peeled, cored and cut into small cubes
- sprinkle of sugar

1 Heat the oil in a large pan, add the onion and fry for 5 mins. Add the garlic and squash, and cook for 5 mins more. Stir in the madeira, stock and chopped sage, then cover and simmer for 20 mins until the squash is tender.

2 Blitz with a hand blender until smooth. Allow to cool in the pan, then chill until ready to serve. Will keep for 2 days or freeze for 3 months. For the crispy sage, heat some oil (a depth of 2cm) in a small pan, then drop in the sage leaves until they are crisp – you will need to do this in batches. Drain on kitchen paper.

3 Just before serving, reheat the soup in a pan. The texture should be quite thick and velvety.

4 For the apple croutons, heat some oil in a large pan, add the apple and fry until starting to soften. Sprinkle with the sugar and stir until lightly caramelised. To serve, ladle the soup into small bowls and top with the apple, sage and a grinding of black pepper.

· ·
GOOD TO KNOW: Vegan
PER SERVING kcal 231, fat 7g, saturates 1g, carbs 31g, sugars 20g, fibre 8g, protein 4g, salt 0.4g

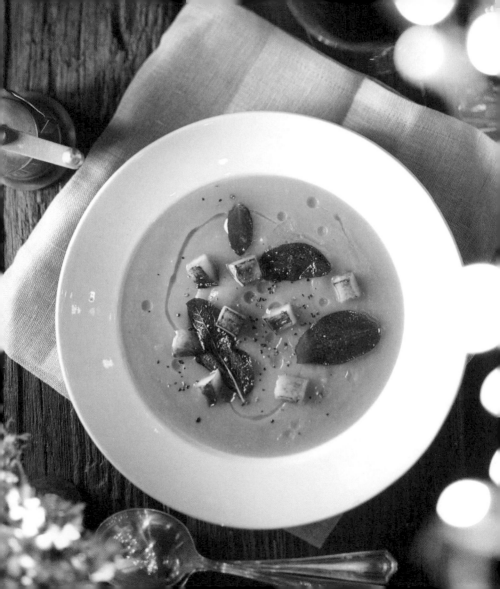

Indian winter soup

Freeze the leftovers for a hearty, spicy soup anytime.

PREP 15 mins COOK 30 mins   4-6

- 100g pearl barley
- 2 tbsp vegetable oil
- ½ tsp brown mustard seeds
- 1 tsp cumin seeds
- 2 green chillies, deseeded and finely chopped
- 2 cloves
- 1 cinnamon stick
- ½ tsp ground turmeric
- 1 large onion, chopped
- 2 garlic cloves, chopped
- 600g mixed root vegetables or squash, chopped
- 1 tsp paprika
- 1 tsp ground coriander
- 225g red lentils
- 2 tomatoes, chopped
- small bunch coriander, chopped
- 1 tsp grated ginger
- 1 tsp lemon juice

1 Rinse the pearl barley and cook following pack instructions. When it is tender, drain and set aside. Meanwhile, heat the oil in a deep, heavy-bottomed pan. Fry the mustard seeds, cumin seeds, chillies, cloves, cinnamon and turmeric until fragrant and the seeds start to crackle. Tip in the onion and garlic, then cook for 5-8 mins until soft. Stir in the vegetables and mix thoroughly, making sure they are fully coated with the oil and spices. Sprinkle in the paprika, ground coriander and seasoning, and stir again.

2 Add the lentils, pearl barley, tomatoes and 1.7 litres water. Bring to the boil then turn down and simmer until the vegetables are tender. When the lentils are almost cooked, stir in the chopped coriander, ginger and lemon juice.

GOOD TO KNOW: Vegan
PER SERVING kcal 445, fat 8g, saturates 1g, carbs 80g, sugars 13g, fibre 8g, protein 19g, salt 0.14g

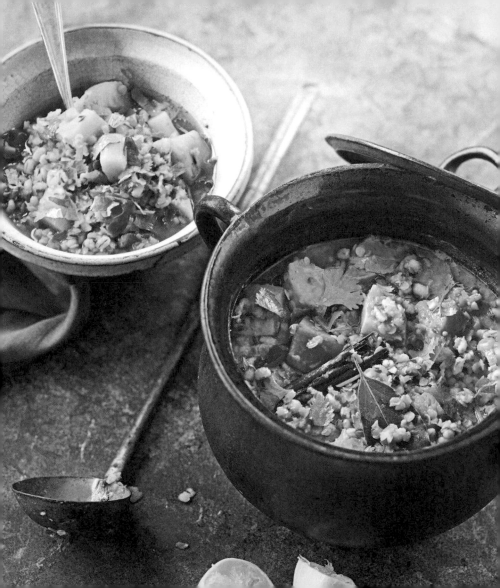

Japanese tofu noodle bowl

This satisfying noodle dish is the perfect spring lunch.

🕐 PREP 15 mins plus marinating COOK 15 mins 🍽 4

- 3 tbsp tamari or dark soy sauce
- 2 tbsp seasoned rice vinegar
- 1 tbsp mirin
- 200g firm tofu, drained, patted dry and cut into 8 cubes
- cornflour, for coating
- sunflower oil, for frying
- 1 bunch asparagus, base of stalks snapped off, cut diagonally into about 4 pieces
- 50g fresh or frozen edamame beans
- 50g frozen peas
- small piece ginger, grated
- 400g pack straight-to-wok udon noodles
- coriander leaves, to garnish
- chilli oil, to serve

1 Combine the tamari or soy sauce, vinegar and mirin in a shallow bowl and stir. Place the tofu in the marinade and turn to coat. Leave to marinate for at least 30 mins. (If marinating for several hours, keep in the fridge.)

2 When ready to cook, scatter the cornflour over a plate. Remove the tofu from the marinade, reserving the marinade, and roll in the cornflour to coat all sides. Heat a frying pan over a medium heat and add enough sunflower oil to cover the base of the pan. Fry the tofu, turning occasionally, until golden and crisp all over. Drain on kitchen paper, then keep warm in a low oven.

3 Place 1 litre of water to the boil in a saucepan with the reserved marinade. Add asparagus, edamame beans, peas, ginger and noodles and return to the boil. Simmer until the vegetables are tender, about 3-4 mins. Divide into 4 bowls and place 2 tofu cubes in each. Top with coriander leaves and serve drizzled with a little of the chilli oil.

GOOD TO KNOW: Vegan
PER SERVING kcal 478, fat 8g, saturates 1g, carbs 87g, sugars 6g, fibre 3g, protein 20g, salt 5.02g

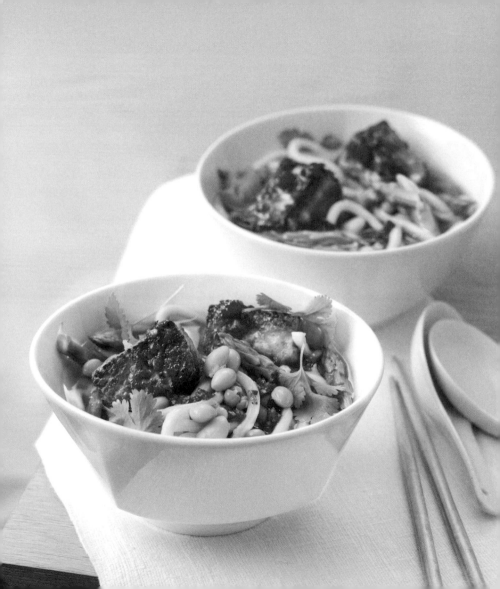

Moroccan spiced cauliflower & almond soup

A smooth, spicy meal in a bowl.

PREP 5 mins COOK 25 mins   4

- 1 large cauliflower
- ½ tsp each ground cinnamon, cumin and coriander
- 2 tbsp harissa paste, plus extra to drizzle
- 2 tbsp olive oil
- 1 litre hot vegetable stock
- 50g toasted flaked almonds, plus extra to serve

Cut the cauliflower into small florets. Fry the ground cinnamon, cumin and coriander and the harissa paste in the olive oil for 2 mins in a large pan. Add the cauliflower, stock and almonds. Cover and cook for 20 mins until the cauliflower is tender. Blend the soup until smooth, then serve with an extra drizzle of harissa and a sprinkle of toasted almonds.

GOOD TO KNOW: Vegan
PER SERVING kcal 200, fat 16g, saturates 2g, carbs 8g, sugars 3g, fibre 3g, protein 8g, salt 2.7g

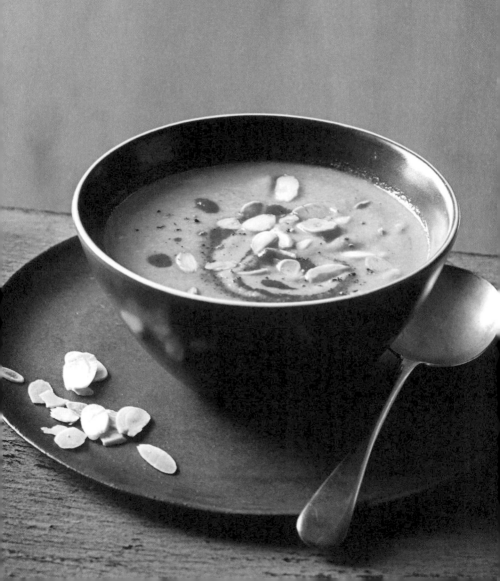

Bean & barley soup

Instead of scattering over grated cheese at the end, why not try mixing 3 tsp ground almonds with 1 tsp nutritional yeast and a pinch of salt for a cheesy vegan topping.

🕐 PREP 5 mins COOK 1 hr 🥧 4

- 2 tbsp vegetable oil
- 1 large onion, finely chopped
- 1 fennel bulb, quartered, cored and sliced
- 5 garlic cloves, crushed
- 400g can chickpeas, drained and rinsed
- 2 x 400g cans chopped tomatoes
- 600ml vegetable stock
- 250g pearl barley
- 215g can butter beans, drained and rinsed
- 100g pack baby spinach leaves
- grated hard cheese, to serve (optional)

1 Heat the oil in a saucepan over a medium heat, add the onion, fennel and garlic, and cook until softened and just beginning to brown, about 10-12 mins.

2 Mash half the chickpeas and add to the pan with the tomatoes, stock and barley. Top up with a can of water and bring to the boil, then reduce the heat and simmer, covered, for 45 mins or until the barley is tender. Add another can of water if the liquid has significantly reduced.

3 Add the remaining chickpeas and the butter beans to the soup. After a few mins, stir in the spinach and cook until wilted, about 1 min. Season and serve scattered with cheese.

GOOD TO KNOW: *Vegetarian*
PER SERVING kcal 488, fat 9g, saturates 1g, carbs 78g, sugars 11g, fibre 12g, protein 16g, salt 1.4g

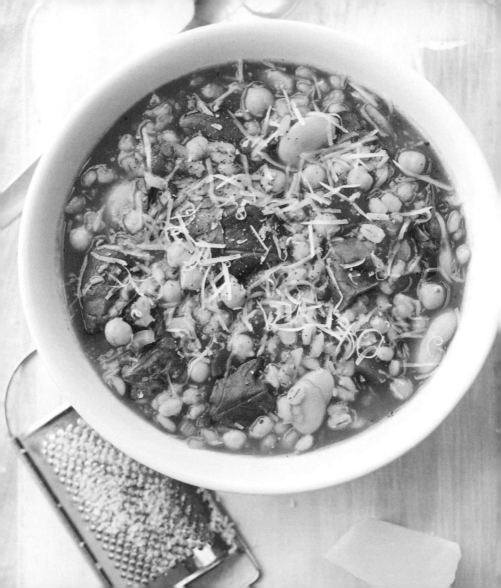

Veggie wholewheat pot noodle

Perk up your packed-lunch with this homemade noodle pot.

🕐 PREP 15 mins COOK 10 mins 🍽 2

- 100g wholewheat noodles
- 2 tsp groundnut oil
- 1 red pepper, cut into fine strips
- ½ large courgette, cut into matchsticks
- 50g frozen shelled edamame beans
- 25g beansprouts
- 1 carrot, peeled and cut into matchsticks
- handful baby spinach
- 2-4 tbsp crispy onions from a tub
- 2 tbsp roughly chopped coriander

FOR THE DRESSING
- 1 tbsp sesame oil
- 2 tbsp yuzu juice (find it at souschef.com or 2 limes, juiced)
- 1 garlic clove, finely chopped
- 1 red chilli, deseeded andfinely chopped
- 1 tsp grated ginger

1 Fill a large saucepan with water and bring to the boil. Add the noodles and cook for 3-5 mins or until tender. Drain and leave to cool.

2 Place a large non-stick pan (or wok) over a medium-high heat and add the groundnut oil. When hot, add the red pepper and cook for 2-3 mins until slightly softened. Add the courgette and edamame, and cook for a further 1-2 mins. Remove from the heat, transfer to a bowl and allow to cool.

3 Whisk together the dressing ingredients in a small bowl, or 2 jars if taking to work, then season. Divide the noodles between 2 jars or plastic containers and top with the cooled vegetables, beansprouts, carrot, spinach, crispy onions and coriander. Add the dressing just before eating.

GOOD TO KNOW: Vegan
PER SERVING kcal 369, fat 11g, saturates 2g, carbs 51g, sugars 13g, fibre 9g, protein 12g, salt 1g

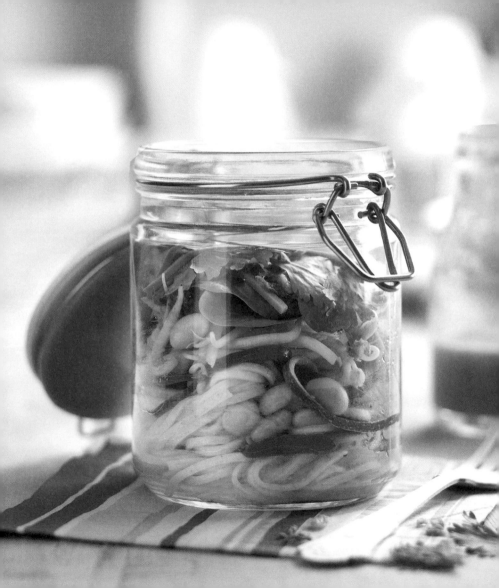

Thai pumpkin soup

. . . .

Autumn veg pairs beautifully with fragrant Thai spices and creamy coconut.

🕐 PREP 25 mins COOK 50 mins 🥧 6

- 1½kg pumpkin or squash, peeled and roughly chopped
- 4 tsp sunflower oil
- 1 onion, sliced
- 1 tbsp grated ginger
- 1 lemongrass, bashed a little
- 3-4 tbsp Thai red curry paste
- 400ml can coconut milk
- 850ml vegetable stock
- lime juice and sugar, for seasoning
- 1 red chilli, sliced, to serve (optional)

1 Heat oven to 200C/180C fan/gas 6. Toss the pumpkin or squash in a roasting tin with half the oil and seasoning, then roast for 30 mins until golden and tender.

2 Meanwhile, put the remaining oil in a pan with the onion, ginger and lemongrass. Gently cook for 8-10 mins until softened. Stir in the curry paste for 1 min, followed by the roasted pumpkin, all but 3 tbsp of the coconut milk and the stock. Bring to a simmer, cook for 5 mins, then fish out the lemongrass. Cool for a few mins, then whizz until smooth with a stick blender or in a large blender in batches. Return to the pan to heat through, seasoning with salt, pepper, lime juice and sugar, if it needs it. Serve drizzled with the remaining coconut milk and scattered with chilli, if you like.

. . . .

GOOD TO KNOW: Vegan
PER SERVING kcal 192, fat 15g, saturates 10g, carbs 11g, sugars 9g, fibre 4g, protein 4g, salt 0.94g

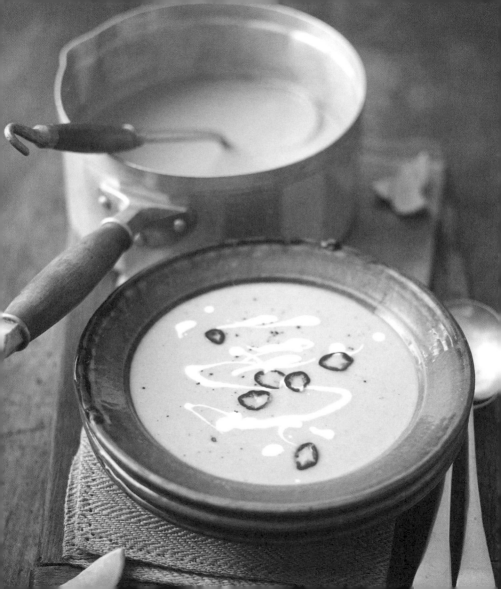

Avocado with tamari & ginger dressing

Avoid an afternoon slump with this quick, easy and tasty snack. Tamari is similar to soy sauce but it's richer and less salty making it delicious as a dip or dressing.

🕐 PREP 5 mins   🍴 2

- 1 small garlic clove, shredded
- ½ tsp shredded ginger
- 1 tsp tamari
- 2 tsp lemon juice
- 1 avocado

Mix the garlic, ginger, tamari and lemon juice in a small bowl. Dilute with 1-2 tsp water. Cut the avocado in half and destone, then spoon in the dressing and eat with a teaspoon.

GOOD TO KNOW: Vegan
PER SERVING kcal 148, fat 14g, saturates 3g, carbs 2g, sugars 1g, fibre 3g, protein 2g, salt 0.4g

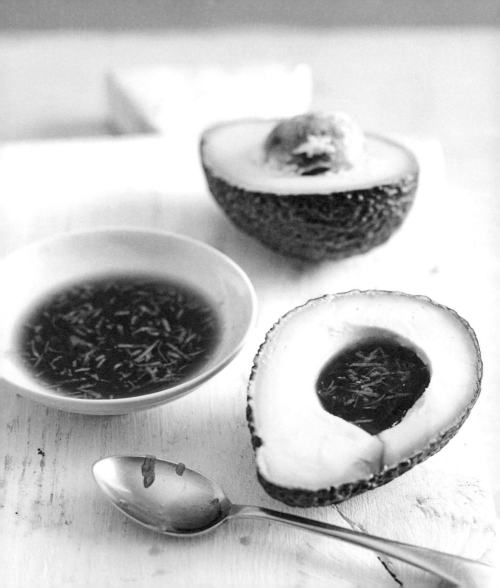

Spicy roast chickpeas

. . . .

A great alternative to peanuts or crisps – simply spice, roast and serve with drinks!

🕓 PREP 5 mins COOK 35 mins   🍽 3-4

- 400g can chickpeas, drained
- 1 tsp extra virgin rapeseed oil
- 1 tsp smoked paprika
- 1 tsp ground cumin
- 1 tsp ground coriander

Heat oven to 180C/160C fan/gas 4. Tip the chickpeas into a bowl and toss with the rapeseed oil, smoked paprika, cumin and coriander. Toss well until the chickpeas are well coated, then tip out onto a baking tray and bake for 35 mins, moving them around the tray halfway through so they dry out evenly and are crunchy. Leave to cool, then store in an airtight container.

. . . .

GOOD TO KNOW: Vegan
PER SERVING kcal 115, fat 3g, saturates 0.3g, carbs 12g, sugars 0.4g, fibre 5g, protein 6g, salt 0g

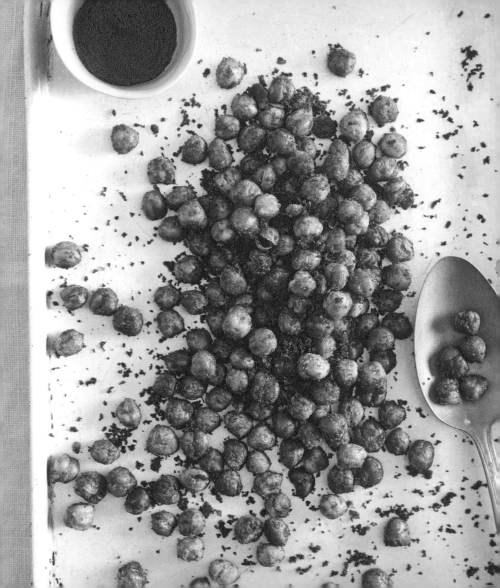

Cinnamon cashew spread with apple slices

· · · · · · · · · · · · · · · · · · · ·

A no-cook handy snack with only five ingredients.

🕐 PREP 10 mins   🥧 2

- 50g unroasted cashew nuts
- 1 tbsp coconut oil
- ½ tsp ground cinnamon
- 2 apples, sliced straight across into rounds
- 2 generous lemon wedges, for squeezing over

Pour boiling water over the cashew nuts in a small bowl to cover, and leave for 2-3 mins so they soften a little. Drain, then return to the bowl. Add the coconut oil and cinnamon and blitz with a stick blender to chop the nuts into a rough paste. Serve with the apples slices and lemon wedges.

· ·
GOOD TO KNOW: Vegan
PER SERVING kcal 239, fat 18g, saturates 7g, carbs 12g, sugars 9g, fibre 3g, protein 6g, salt 0g

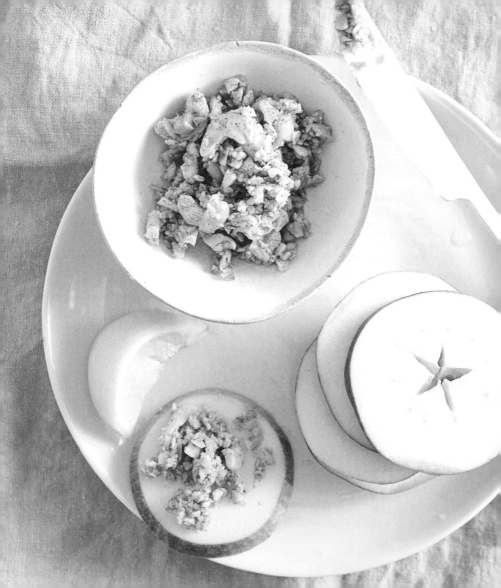

Carrot & cumin houmous with swirled harissa

Great with flatbreads and crunchy vegetables –it travels well so perfect for a picnic.

PREP 5 mins COOK 40 mins | 8

- 600g carrots
- 2 tbsp olive oil
- 1 tsp cumin seeds
- 1 garlic bulb, broken into cloves
- juice of 1 lemon
- 120ml extra virgin olive oil
- 400g can chickpeas, drained and rinsed
- rose harissa, to serve
- flatbreads, to serve

1 Heat oven to 200C/180C fan/gas 6. Cut the carrots into chunks and toss with the olive oil, cumin seeds and garlic bulb. Spread onto a baking tray and roast in the oven for 40 mins or until caramelised.

2 Squeeze the garlic cloves out of their skins and tip into a food processor with the carrots, lemon juice, extra virgin olive oil, chickpeas and some seasoning. Blitz until smooth. Swirl through some spicy rose harissa and serve with flatbreads

GOOD TO KNOW: Vegan
PER SERVING kcal 239, fat 19g, saturates 3g, carbs 11g, sugars 6g, fibre 5g, protein 3g, salt 0.1g

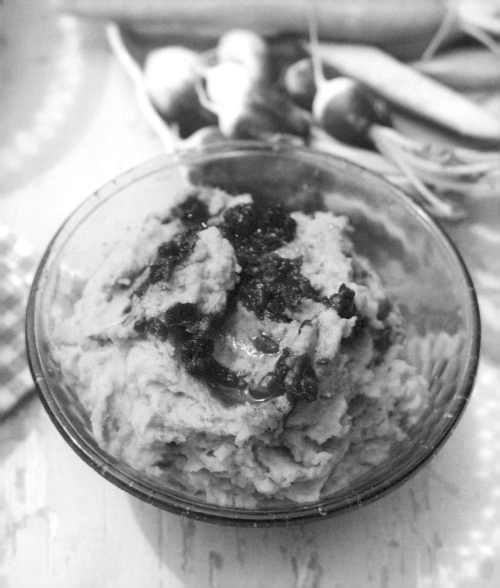

Crushed pea & mint dip with carrot sticks

. . . .

A tablespoon of houmous makes an easy vegan swap for the ricotta in this recipe.

PREP 5 mins 1

- 70g defrosted frozen peas
- 1 tbsp ricotta
- juice of ½ lemon
- handful chopped mint
- 1 carrot, cut into sticks for dipping

In the small bowl of a food processor, blitz the peas with the ricotta, lemon juice, mint and some black pepper. Serve with the carrot sticks.

. . . .
GOOD TO KNOW: Vegetarian
PER SERVING kcal 121, fat 3g, saturates 1g, carbs 15g, sugars 11g, fibre 8g, protein 6g, salt 0.1g

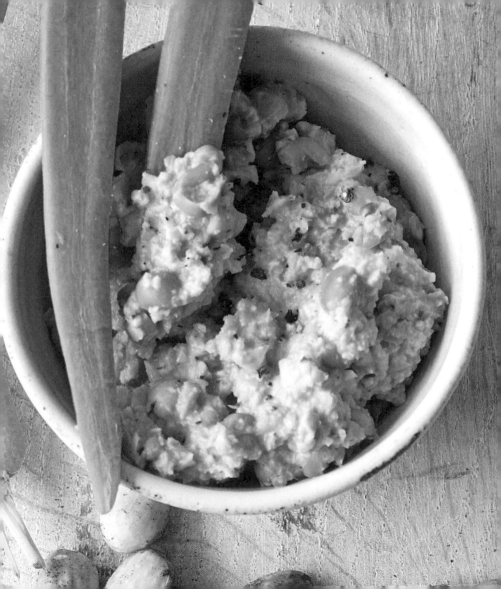

Sweet potato fries

Enjoy these as a snack or as a simple side dish.

 PREP 2 mins COOK 20 mins 1

- 95g sweet potato, cut into fries
- 1 tsp extra virgin rapeseed oil
- ¼ tsp cayenne pepper

Heat oven to 200C/180C fan/ gas 6. Put the sweet potato fries on a baking tray and mix with the rapeseed oil and cayenne pepper. Bake in the oven for 20 mins.

GOOD TO KNOW: Vegan
PER SERVING kcal 147, fat 3g, saturates 0g, carbs 25g, sugars 13g, fibre 4g, protein 1g, salt 0.1g

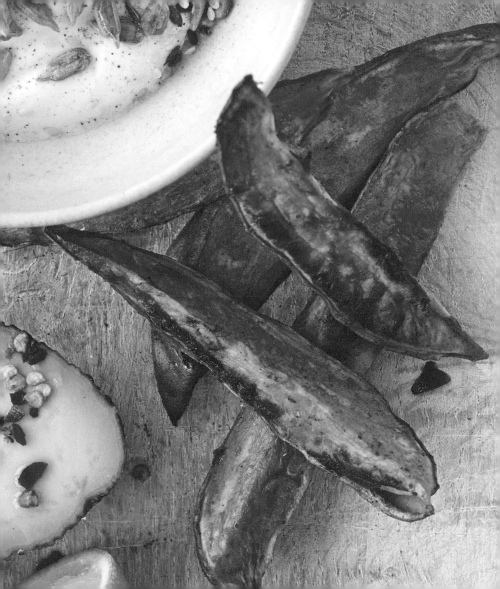

Za'atar croutons

. . . .

Crunchy bites, moreish on their own or serve with smashed avocado or a tahini dip.
Za'atar is a fragrant Middle Eastern spice mix, find it in larger supermarkets or make
your own from our recipe at bbcgoodfood.com

🕐 PREP 5 mins COOK 40 mins 🥧 2

- 2 round pitta breads
- 2 tbsp olive oil
- 1 tbsp za'atar spice mix

1 Heat oven to 110C/90C fan/gas ¼. Put the
  pittas on top of each other on a chopping
  board. With a bread knife, cut them into
  quarters, then cut each quarter in half again
  (so you end up with 16 equal-sized triangles).
2 Add the olive oil, a pinch of salt and the
  za'atar to a small bowl, and stir to combine.
  Using a pastry brush or your fingers, coat the
  pittas on both sides with the mixture, then put
  them on a baking tray and bake in the oven
  for 30-40 mins until crisp.

. . . .
GOOD TO KNOW: Vegan
PER SERVING kcal 304, fat 12g, saturates 2g, carbs 39g, sugars 2g, fibre 2g, protein 8g, salt 0.8g

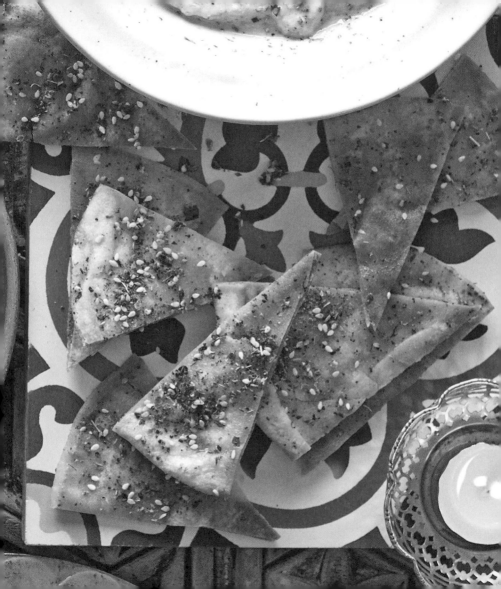

Spinach & sweet potato samosas

A family-friendly snack, packed with veg. For vegans serve just with the mango chutney or add a plain dairy-free yogurt.

🕐 PREP 35 mins COOK 45 mins 🥧 3-4

- 500g sweet potatoes, peeled and chopped
- 1 tbsp vegetable oil, plus extra for brushing
- 2 red onions, 1 chopped, 1 halved and finely sliced
- thumb-sized piece ginger, peeled and finely chopped
- 2 garlic cloves, crushed
- 1 red chilli, finely chopped (optional)
- small bunch coriander, stalks chopped, leaves picked
- 2 tbsp curry paste (we used balti)
- 200g bag spinach, wilted in boiling water and drained
- 2 tsp black onion seeds
- 270g pack filo pastry (6 sheets)
- 150ml pot natural yogurt
- ½ cucumber, cut into ribbons
- mango chutney, to serve

1 Put the sweet potatoes in a bowl and cover with cling film. Microwave for 8 mins or until tender. Soften the chopped onion in a pan with the oil, then add the ginger, garlic, chilli and coriander stalks and cook until fragrant. Add the curry paste, spinach, sweet potato and half the onion seeds. Season and roughly mash, then leave to cool.

2 Brush 2 sheets of pastry with oil and stack together. Cut down the centre to make 2 long strips. Scoop a sixth of the sweet potato mixture onto the top right-hand corner of the filo. Start folding the pastry over on an angle down the length to make a neat triangular parcel. Repeat to make 6 samosas. Heat oven to 200C/180C fan/gas 6 and line a tray with baking parchment.

3 Brush the samosas with oil, add the remaining onion seeds and bake for 25-30 mins. Serve with the yogurt, cucumber, sliced onion, coriander leaves and mango chutney.

GOOD TO KNOW: Vegetarian
PER SERVING kcal 650, fat 13g, saturates 2g, carbs 108g, sugars 36g, fibre 15g, protein 17g, salt 1.5g

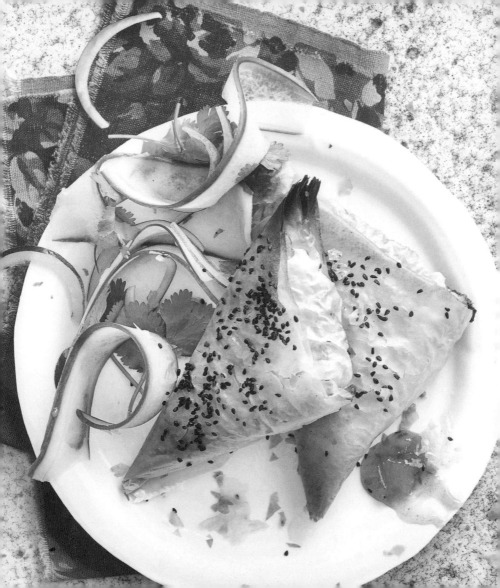

Spiced pea & potato rolls

A filling snack made with storecupboard staples.

🕐 PREP 15 mins COOK 35 mins 🕔 MAKES 4

- 2 tbsp vegetable oil or sunflower oil
- 2 onions, finely sliced
- 300g potatoes, cut into small cubes
- 1 heaped tbsp curry paste
- 140g frozen or fresh peas
- 4 large sheets filo pastry, cut in half
- tomatoes, onion and mango chutney, to serve

1 Heat oven to 220C/200C fan/gas 7. Heat half the oil in a non-stick frying pan. Tip in the onions and cook until soft and golden, about 8-10 mins. Meanwhile, boil the potato cubes for 5 mins, until just tender, then drain. Tip into the softened onions and fry for 2 mins more. Stir in the curry paste and cook for 2 mins. Pop in the peas, plus 1 tbsp water. Cook for 1 min, give everything a good mix and season. Tip into a bowl to allow to cool slightly.

2 Brush half the filo half-sheets with some of the remaining oil, then lay the remaining sheets on top so you have 4 x double layers. Spoon a quarter of the potato mix along one edge of each, leaving a bit of space at each end. Fold in the ends t,hen roll up to seal. Place seam-side down on a baking sheet, brush with the remaining oil and bake for 20 mins, or until crisp. Serve warm with a dollop of mango chutney and a tomato & onion salad, if you like.

GOOD TO KNOW: Vegan
PER SERVING kcal 240, fat 8g, saturates 1g, carbs 37g, sugars 6g, fibre 4g, protein 7g, salt 0.46g

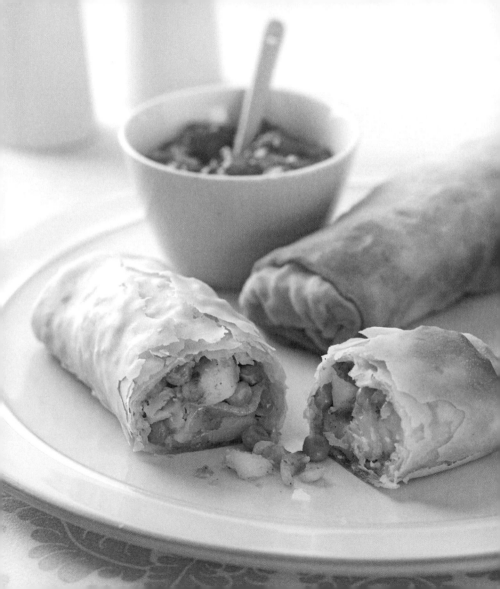

Yakitori corn pops

A fun snack or casual starter for a crowd.

🕐 PREP 15 mins COOK 20 mins 🕐 MAKES 8-12

- 2 fresh corn cobs, leaves and threads peeled away
- about 150ml good yakitori sauce (or see recipe in tip, below)
- 1 tbsp sunflower oil
- 8-12 wooden chopsticks or short skewers
- 3 tbsp toasted sesame seeds

1 Put the corn cobs in a microwaveable dish with about 1cm water. Cover with cling film, poke a couple of holes through and microwave for 10 mins on high until tender. When cool enough to handle, trim the rounded ends and cut the rest into 3-5cm chunks. Mix 1 tbsp yakitori sauce with the oil and brush all over the corn.

2 Heat a griddle pan or barbecue and sear the corn on all sides until starting to char. Lift into a bowl, dip into the remaining yakitori sauce and toss to coat. Add a stick to each – like a lollipop – then dip each corn pop into the sesame seeds to coat before eating.

TIP: For a homemade yakitori sauce, mix 1 tbsp cornflour with 1 tbsp sake to a paste. Put 2 more tbsp sake, 125ml light soy sauce, 4 tbsp mirin and 2 tsp golden caster sugar in a small saucepan, whisk in the cornflour and heat until the sugar has melted and sauce thickened, then cool before serving.

GOOD TO KNOW: *Vegan*
PER SERVING *kcal 55, fat 2g, saturates 0g, carbs 6g, sugars 2g, fibre 1g, protein 1g, salt 1.2g*

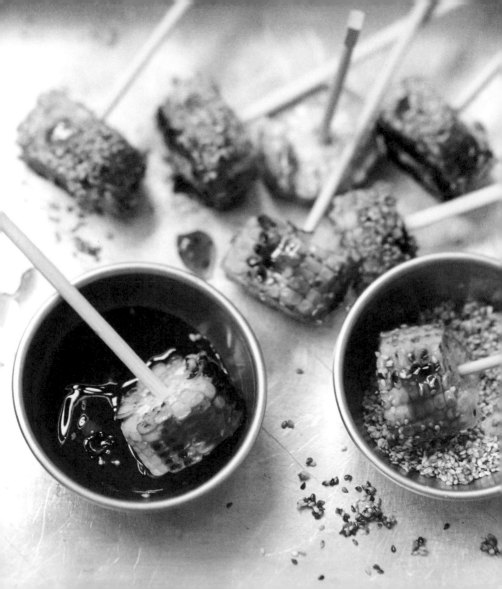

Choc-orange energy boosters

A high-energy snack. Try coating the finished boosters in dark chocolate for a rich after-dinner treat.

🕐 PREP 15 mins   🗓 MAKES about 18

- 100g pitted Medjool dates
- 100g pecan nuts
- 50g pumpkin seeds
- 50g rolled oats
- 4 tbsp cacao powder or unsweetened cocoa
- 2 heaped tbsp almond butter
- zest and juice of 1 orange

Place all the ingredients and 3 tbsp orange juice in a food processor. Blitz until chopped and starting to clump together. If it's a bit dry, add a drop more orange juice. Roll the mixture into walnut-sized balls with lightly oiled hands. Pop 2 or 3 into a lunchbox for a snack. Keeps in a sealed container for 2 weeks in the fridge.

GOOD TO KNOW: Vegan
PER SERVING kcal 99, fat 6g, saturates 1g, carbs 7g, sugars 4g, fibre 2g, protein 3g, salt 0g

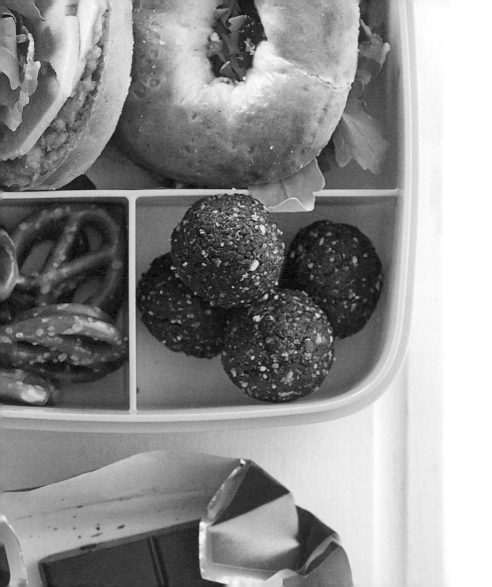

Crunchy bulghar salad

The edamame beans and almonds provide tasty sources of protein in this vibrant summer salad.

PREP 10 mins COOK 15 mins 4

- 200g bulghar wheat
- 150g frozen shelled edamame beans
- 2 Romano peppers, sliced into rounds, seeds removed
- 150g radishes, finely sliced
- 75g whole blanched almonds
- small bunch mint, finely chopped
- small bunch parsley, finely chopped
- 2 oranges
- 3 tbsp extra virgin olive oil

1 Cook the bulghar following pack instructions, then drain and tip into a large serving bowl to cool. Meanwhile, put the edamame beans in a small bowl, pour over boiling water, leave for 1 min, then drain. Put in a serving bowl with the peppers, radishes, almonds, mint and parsley.

2 Peel one orange, carefully cut away the segments and add to the bowl. Squeeze the juice of the other into a jam jar with the oil. Season well and shake to emulsify. Pour over the salad, toss well and serve

GOOD TO KNOW: *Vegan*
PER SERVING kcal 483, fat 22g, saturates 2g, carbs 50g, sugars 11g, fibre 9g, protein 17g, salt 0g

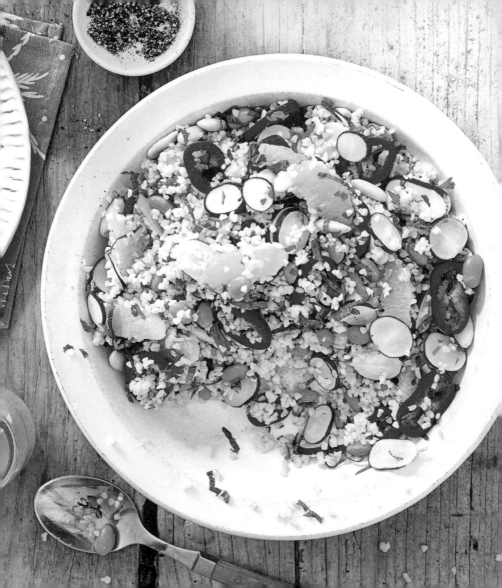

Roasted cauli-broc bowl

Cook the veg the night before, then the following day assemble in 10 minutes for a simple al-desko lunch.

PREP 10 mins COOK 30 mins   2

- 400g pack cauliflower and broccoli florets
- 2 tbsp olive oil
- 250g ready-to-eat quinoa
- 2 cooked beetroots, cubed
- large handful baby spinach
- 10 walnuts, toasted and chopped
- 2 tbsp tahini
- 3 tbsp houmous
- 1 lemon, ½ juiced, ½ cut into wedges

1 Heat oven to 200C/180C fan/gas 6. Put the cauliflower and broccoli in a large roasting tin with the oil and a sprinkle of flaky sea salt. Roast for 25-30 mins until browned and cooked. Leave to cool completely.

2 Build each bowl by putting half the quinoa in each. Lay the cubes of beetroot on top, followed by the spinach, cauliflower, broccoli and walnuts. Combine the tahini, houmous, lemon juice and 1 tbsp water in a small pot. Before eating, coat in the dressing. Serve with the lemon wedges.

GOOD TO KNOW: Vegan
PER SERVING kcal 533, fat 37g, saturates 4g, carbs 28g, sugars 6g, fibre 10g, protein 16g, salt 0.8g

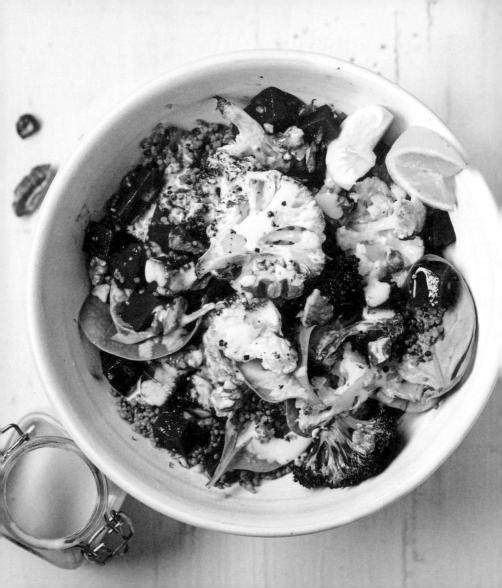

Sesame stir-fry wrap

A refreshing lunch that's speedy to prepare and pack for work on busy mornings.

🕐 PREP 5 mins   👤 1

- 2 tbsp tahini
- juice ½ lemon
- 1 large wholemeal tortilla wrap
- ½ x 265g pack stir-fry vegetables
- ½ tbsp sesame seeds

Mix the tahini with the lemon juice and 1 tbsp water to form a paste. Spread on the base of the wholemeal tortilla wrap with some seasoning. Scatter over the stir-fry vegetables and sesame seeds. Roll up in a tight wrap and halve to serve.

GOOD TO KNOW: Vegan
PER SERVING kcal 511, fat 32g, saturates 6g, carbs 32g, sugars 6g, fibre 0g, protein 0g, salt 0g

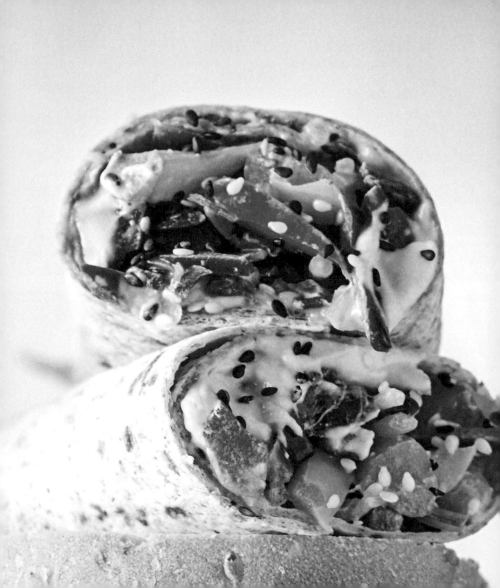

Keep it green sandwich

The chickpeas make this much more filling than your usual salad sarnie.

🕐 PREP 10 mins 🍽 1

- 25g curly kale
- ½ tbsp sesame oil
- ½ tbsp tamari
- 1 small avocado
- juice 1 small lime
- 40g drained canned chickpeas
- 2 slices rye bread
- ½ tsp paprika

Massage the curly kale in the sesame oil and tamari for a few mins until softened, then set aside. Smash the avocado with a fork in a bowl with the lime juice, chickpeas and some seasoning. Spread across 1 slice of rye, lay the kale on top and sprinkle with the paprika. Top with another slice of rye and halve.

GOOD TO KNOW: Vegan
PER SERVING kcal 443, fat 27g, saturates 5g, carbs 32g, sugars 2g, fibre 10g, protein 11g, salt 1.8g

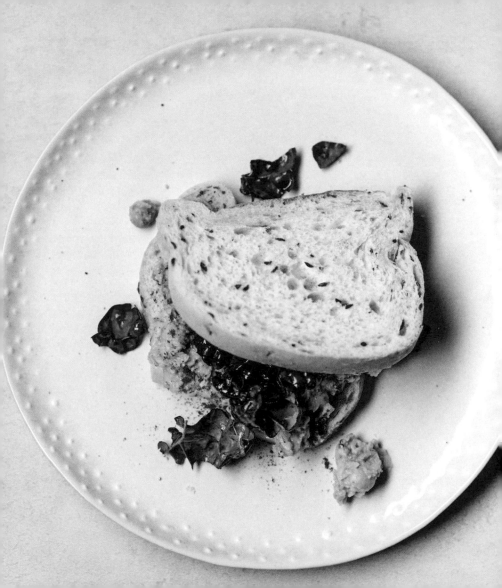

California quinoa & avocado salad

This smart, modern lunch is easily doubled if you've got guests for lunch.

PREP 10 mins COOK 30 mins   2

- 250g butternut squash, chopped
- 2 tbsp olive oil
- 120g pack thin-stemmed broccoli, roughly chopped
- 250g pouch cooked quinoa
- small handful coriander, chopped
- small handful mint, chopped
- 4 spring onions, finely sliced
- 50g pomegranate seeds
- 20g pistachios, roughly chopped
- 1 small ripe avocado, sliced
- juice ½ lemon
- handful alfalfa sprouts

FOR THE DRESSING

- 1 tbsp tahini
- ½ ripe avocado, chopped
- small handful coriander leaves
- small handful mint leaves
- zest and juice ½ lemon
- 2 tsp maple syrup

1 Heat oven to 200C/180C fan/gas 6. Line a baking tray with parchment. Tip the butternut squash onto the tray, drizzle with 2 tsp oil and season. Roast for 20 mins, add the broccoli to the tray and drizzle with 1 tsp oil. Season and roast for 10 mins more.

2 For the dressing, put all the ingredients in the small bowl of a food processor, add 1 tbsp water and a pinch of salt. Blitz to make a loose dressing, adding more water if needed.

3 Tip the quinoa into a large bowl. Add the herbs, spring onions, pomegranate seeds, pistachios, roasted veg and remaining oil, season and toss together.

4 Divide the salad and dressing between 2 plates. Squeeze the lemon juice over the avocado, then add to each salad. Top with the sprouts and grind over a little pepper, if you like.

GOOD TO KNOW: Vegan
PER SERVING kcal 740, fat 44g, saturates 6g, carbs 59g, sugars 17g, fibre 17g, protein 18g, salt 0.9g

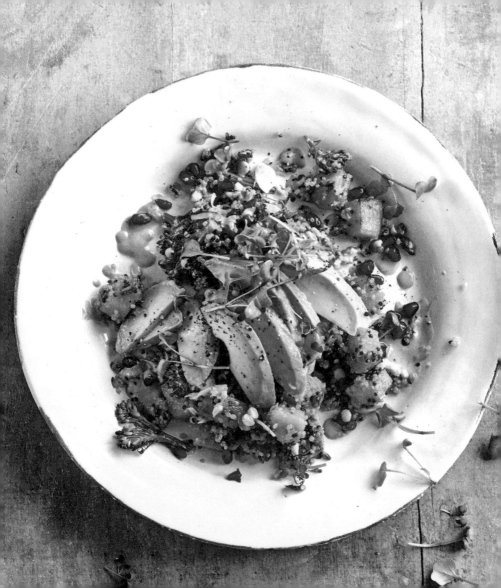

No-cook festival burrito

A filling lunch or hearty brunch that uses ingredients that don't all need to be refrigerated, making it perfect for festivals or camping holidays.

🕐 PREP 30 mins plus soaking 🥧 4

- 100g bulghar wheat
- 120g cherry tomatoes, roughly chopped
- 3 tbsp tahini
- 4 tortilla wraps
- 215g can kidney beans, drained
- 198g can sweetcorn, drained
- 200g smoked tofu (we used Taifun smoked tofu with almonds and sesame seeds)
- 50g grilled red peppers
- 1 avocado, roughly chopped
- 1 lime, quartered
- chilli sauce to serve (optional), we used sriracha

1 Put the bulghar wheat into a bowl and add 100ml of boiling water. Cover and leave to soak for 35-40 mins, then add the tomatoes and season.

2 In a small bowl or cup mix the tahini with 3 tbsp of water to make a smooth and pourable sauce.

3 Lay the tortilla wraps out on plates and divide the bulghar wheat, kidney beans and sweetcorn among them. Crumble the smoked tofu over the top, then add the grilled peppers, avocado pieces and a good drizzle of the tahini sauce, a squeeze of lime and some chilli sauce, if you like.

4 Roll up the wraps to completely enclose the filling inside, pushing down to seal. Serve with extra lime and chilli sauce on the side.

GOOD TO KNOW: Vegan
PER SERVING kcal 524, fat 24g, saturates 5g, carbs 47g, sugars 5g, fibre 13g, protein 23g, salt 1.5g

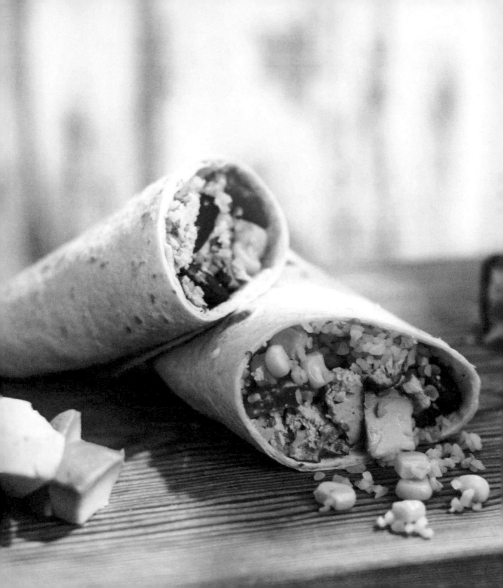

Spice-crusted tofu with kumquat radish salad

· · · · · · · · · · · · · · · · · · · ·

Firm tofu is drier than the silken type making it a good alternative to meat as it holds together much better when frying.

🕐 PREP 10 mins COOK 5 mins 🍽 2

- 200g firm tofu
- 2 tbsp sesame seeds
- 1 tbsp Japanese shichimi togarashi spice mix (available from souschef.co.uk)
- ½ tbsp cornflour
- 1 tbsp sesame oil
- 1 tbsp vegetable oil
- 200g Tenderstem broccoli
- 100g sugar snap peas
- 4 radishes, thinly sliced
- 2 spring onions, finely chopped
- 3 kumquats, thinly sliced

FOR THE DRESSING

- 2 tbsp low-salt Japanese soy sauce
- 2 tbsp yuzu juice (or 1 tbsp each lime and grapefruit juice)
- 1 tsp golden caster sugar
- 1 small shallot, finely diced
- 1 tsp grated ginger

1 Slice the tofu in half, wrap well in kitchen paper and put on a plate. Place a heavy frying pan on top to squeeze the water out of it. Change the paper a few times until the tofu feels dry, then cut into chunky slices. Mix together the sesame seeds, Japanese spice mix and cornflour in a bowl. Sprinkle over the tofu until well coated. Set aside.

2 In a small bowl, mix the dressing ingredients together and set aside. Bring a pan of water to the boil for the vegetables and heat the 2 oils in a large frying pan. When the frying pan is very hot, add the tofu and fry for 1 min or so on each side until nicely browned. Repeat until you have done them all.

3 When the water is boiling, cook the broccoli and sugar snap peas for 2-3 mins. Drain and divide between 2 large shallow bowls or plates. Top with the tofu and drizzle over the dressing. Scatter the radishes, spring onions and kumquats on top.

· ·

GOOD TO KNOW: Vegan
PER SERVING kcal 528, fat 33g, saturates 5g, carbs 24g, sugars 13g, fibre 12g, protein 27g, salt 1.9g

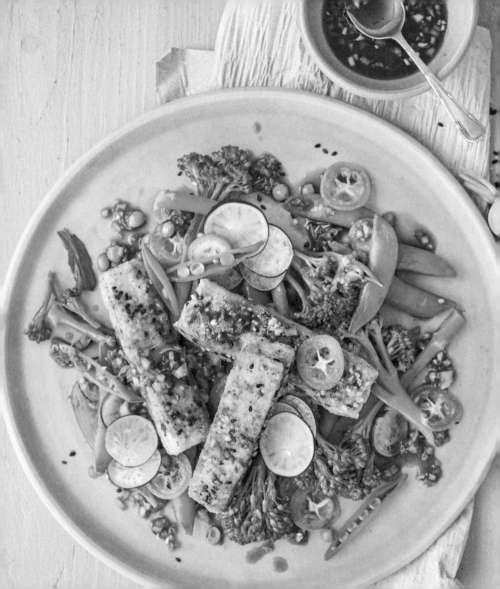

Green rice with beetroot & apple salsa

An easy, flavour-packed lunch dish.

PREP 10 mins COOK 25 mins 2

FOR THE RICE
- 85g brown basmati rice
- 140g fine green beans
- ½ small cucumber, finely diced
- ½ bunch spring onions (about 5), sliced
- ⅓ pack mint, chopped, plus extra leaves to serve
- juice ½ lemon

FOR THE SALSA
- 1 cooked beetroot, diced
- 1 small apple, cored and diced
- 1 small red onion, finely chopped
- 25g walnut halves, roughly broken
- 1 tbsp balsamic vinegar

1 Boil the rice for 20 mins, then add the green beans and cook 5 mins more until both are just tender. Drain and leave to cool slightly before stirring in the cucumber, spring onions, mint and lemon juice.

2 Meanwhile, stir all the salsa ingredients together. Spoon the rice onto plates and serve with the salsa, scattered with a few extra mint leaves.

GOOD TO KNOW: Vegan
PER SERVING kcal 332, fat 11g, saturates 1g, carbs 45g, sugars 12g, fibre 8g, protein 10g, salt 0.1g

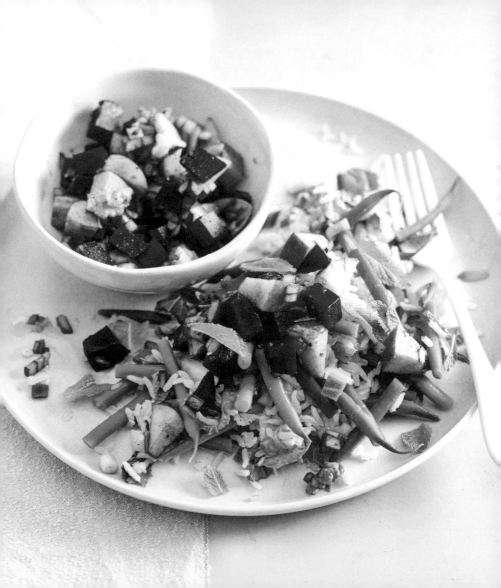

Avocado panzanella

A colourful summer lunch or vibrant buffet platter.

🕐 PREP 20 mins   🍰 4

- 800g mix of ripe tomatoes
- 1 garlic clove, crushed
- 1½ tbsp capers, drained and rinsed
- 1 ripe avocado, stoned, peeled and chopped
- 1 small red onion, very thinly sliced
- 175g ciabatta or crusty loaf
- 4 tbsp extra virgin olive oil
- 2 tbsp red wine vinegar
- small handful basil leaves

1 Halve or roughly chop the tomatoes (depending on size) and put them in a bowl. Season well and add the garlic, capers, avocado and onion, and mix well. Set aside for 10 mins.

2 Meanwhile, tear or slice the ciabatta into 3cm chunks and place in a large serving bowl or on a platter. Drizzle with half the olive oil, half the vinegar and add some seasoning. When you are ready to serve, pour over the tomatoes and any juices. Scatter with the basil leaves and drizzle over the remaining olive oil and vinegar. Give it a final stir and serve immediately.

GOOD TO KNOW: Vegan
PER SERVING kcal 332, fat 21g, saturates 4g, carbs 30g, sugars 8g, fibre 6g, protein 7g, salt 0.9g

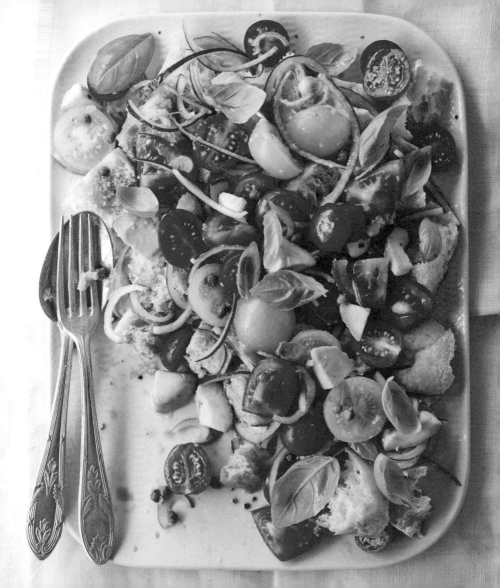

Crispy sweet potatoes with chickpeas & tahini yogurt

· ·

Your new favourite vegetarian barbecue dish. To make this recipe vegan rather than veggie, swap the yogurt for a dairy-free alternative.

🕐 PREP 20 mins COOK 1 hr 🍽 4

- 4 medium sweet potatoes
- 4 tbsp olive oil
- 1 large garlic clove, crushed
- 1 banana shallot, finely chopped
- 400g can chickpeas, drained
- 75g baby spinach leaves
- small bunch dill, finely chopped
- zest and juice 1 lemon

FOR THE TAHINI YOGURT
- 60g Greek yogurt
- 2 tbsp tahini
- 20g pine nuts, toasted
- 110g pomegranate seeds

1 Wrap the potatoes in foil and put on the hot barbecue coals for 35-45 mins or until cooked through. (Alternatively, bake at 200C/180C fan/gas 6 for 45 mins-1 hr, then grill for 3 mins until the skin is blackened and crispy.)

2 Heat 1 tbsp olive oil in a frying pan over a medium heat. Add the garlic and shallot and fry for 2-3 mins, then stir in the chickpeas. Warm through for 1 min, then add the spinach until wilted, followed by the dill.

3 In a bowl, whisk together the lemon juice, zest and remaining olive oil. Season to taste and stir into the chickpea mixture. Gently mash with a potato masher until the chickpeas are slightly crushed. Mix together the yogurt and tahini in another bowl and season to taste.

4 Split the potatoes open lengthways. Fill with the bean mixture, drizzle over the tahini yogurt and top with the pine nuts and pomegranate seeds.

· ·

GOOD TO KNOW: Vegetarian
PER SERVING kcal 535, fat 23g, saturates 4g, carbs 63g, sugars 31g, fibre 13g, protein 12g, salt 0.3g

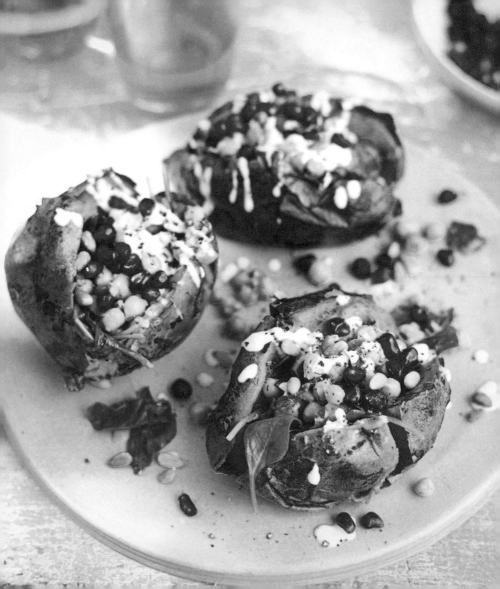

Veggie tahini lentils

Pre-cooked lentils are useful addition to your storecupboard as they're great for making speedy weeknight suppers.

🕐 PREP 10 mins COOK 10 mins 🍽 4

- 50g tahini
- zest and juice 1 lemon
- 2 tbsp olive oil
- 1 red onion, thinly sliced
- 1 garlic clove, crushed
- 1 yellow pepper, thinly sliced
- 200g green beans, trimmed
- 1 courgette, sliced into half moons
- 100g shredded kale
- 250g pack pre-cooked Puy lentils

1 In a jug, mix the tahini with the zest and juice of the lemon and 50ml of cold water to make a runny dressing. Season with salt and pepper to taste, then set aside.

2 Heat the oil in a wok or large frying pan over a medium-high heat. Add the red onion, along with a pinch of salt, and fry for 2 mins until starting to soften and colour. Add the garlic, pepper, green beans and courgette and fry for 5 min, stirring frequently.

3 Tip in the shredded kale, lentils and the tahini dressing. Keep the pan on the heat for a couple of mins, stirring everything together until the kale is wilted and it's all coated in the creamy dressing

GOOD TO KNOW: Vegan
PER SERVING kcal 293, fat 14g, saturates 2g, carbs 23g, sugars 7g, fibre 10g, protein 13g, salt 0.7g

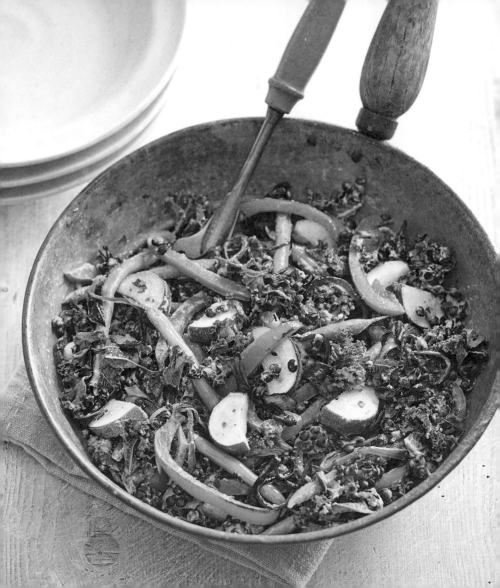

Dukkah-crusted aubergine steaks

Serve these aubergine with a dollop of houmous or dairy-free yogurt on the side instead of the natural yogurt to make them vegan. Dukkah is an Egyptian spice mix, made with hazelnuts, often used with warm bread and olive oil.

🕐 PREP 15 mins COOK 30 mins   🍽 2

- 25g blanched hazelnuts, toasted
- 1½ tsp cumin seeds, toasted
- 1½ tsp fennel seeds, toasted
- large aubergine, trimmed and sliced lengthways into 4 thick steaks
- 2 tbsp olive oil
- juice 1 orange, zest of ½
- 175g couscous
- small pack mint, leaves picked and finely chopped
- 2 tbsp pomegranate seeds
- 50g pot natural yogurt

1 To make the dukkah, lightly crush the hazelnuts, cumin and fennel seeds, and a pinch of salt using a pestle and mortar. Heat oven to 180C/160C fan/gas 4 and heat a griddle pan over a medium heat. Brush the aubergine steaks with 1 tbsp olive oil, griddle for 8-10 mins each side until charred and completely softened, then place on a parchment-lined baking tray. Divide the orange zest among the steaks, then top each with the dukkah. Bake for 5-10 mins until the dukkah looks toasted. Boil the kettle.

2 Put the couscous in a heatproof bowl, add 225ml boiling water and cover with cling film. Leave to stand for 5 mins, then fluff up the couscous with a fork. Mix together the orange juice, remaining olive oil, the mint and some seasoning. Add to the couscous and stir. Divide the couscous between 2 plates, top with the aubergine steaks and sprinkle with the pomegranate seeds. Serve with a dollop of yogurt.

GOOD TO KNOW: *Vegetarian*
PER SERVING kcal 543, fat 24g, saturates 4g, carbs 61g, sugars 16g, fibre 9g, protein 16g, salt 0.2g

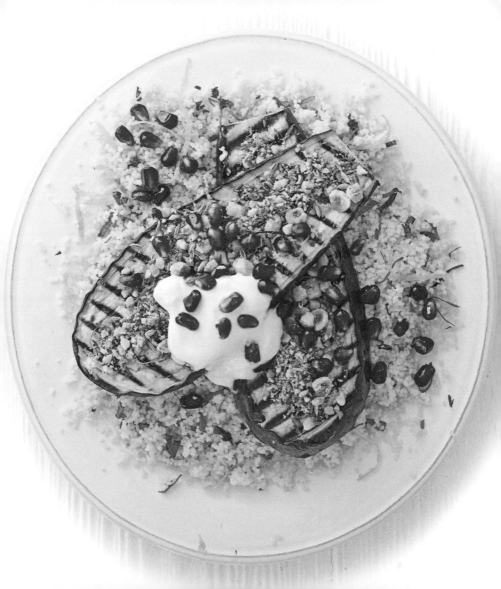

Kidney bean curry

· ·

Adding the water from the can of kidney beans may sound odd but it adds extra flavour and helps creates the smooth texture in the sauce.

🕐 PREP 5 mins COOK 30 mins 🍽 2

- 1 tbsp vegetable oil
- 1 onion, finely chopped
- 2 garlic cloves, finely chopped
- thumb-sized piece ginger, peeled and finely chopped
- 1 small pack coriander, stalks finely chopped, leaves roughly shredded
- 1 tsp ground cumin
- 1 tsp ground paprika
- 2 tsp garam masala
- 400g can chopped tomatoes
- 400g can kidney beans, in water
- cooked basmati rice, to serve

1 Heat the oil in a large frying pan over a low-medium heat. Add the onion and a pinch of salt and cook slowly, stirring occasionally, until softened and just starting to colour. Add the garlic, ginger and coriander stalks and cook for a further 2 mins, until fragrant.

2 Add the spices to the pan and cook for another 1 min, by which point everything should smell aromatic. Tip in the chopped tomatoes and kidney beans in their water, then bring to the boil.

3 Turn down the heat and simmer for 15 mins until the curry is nice and thick. Season to taste, then serve with the basmati rice and the coriander leaves.

· ·
GOOD TO KNOW: Vegan
PER SERVING kcal 282, fat 8g, saturates 1g, carbs 33g, sugars 13g, fibre 14g, protein 13g, salt 0.1g

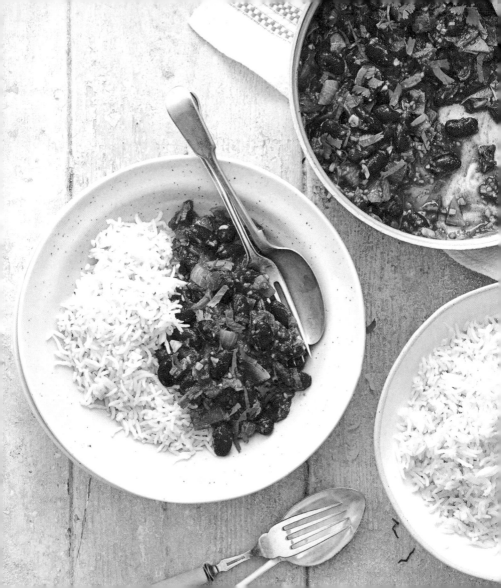

Wholewheat spaghetti & avocado sauce

. . . .

The almonds and avocado make for a creamy, pesto-like sauce. Skip the cheese on the top and serve with extra fresh basil for a totally vegan supper.

⏱ PREP 10 mins COOK 15 mins 🍽 4

- 2 avocados, stoned, peeled and chopped
- zest and juice 1 lemon
- 25g blanched almonds
- 1 garlic clove
- small pack basil
- 300g wholewheat spaghetti
- 25g parmesan, finely grated, to serve (optional)

1 Put the avocados, lemon zest and juice, almonds, garlic and half the basil in a food processor. Blend until smooth, then set aside in the fridge.

2 Cook the spaghetti following pack instructions. Drain and toss in the creamy avocado sauce. Top with the remaining basil leaves and grated parmesan, if using, before serving.

. . . .

GOOD TO KNOW: *Vegetarian*
PER SERVING kcal 435, fat 20g, saturates 3g, carbs 47g, sugars 2g, fibre 10g, protein 13g, salt 0.2g

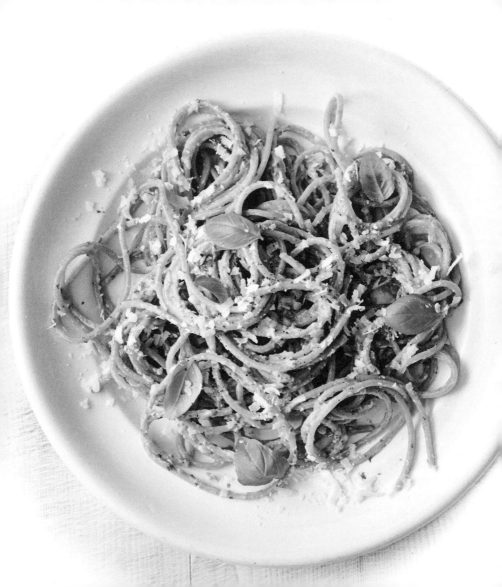

Spicy vegetable pilau with cucumber raita

· ·

Toast the cashews in a dry pan until golden before serving for added oomph.

🕐 PREP 20 mins COOK 30 mins 🍽 2

- 2 garlic cloves
- 1 tbsp extra virgin rapeseed oil
- 1 large onion, sliced
- thumb-sized piece ginger, chopped
- 1 cinnamon stick
- ½ tsp cumin seeds
- seeds from 8 cardamom pods
- 1 tsp ground turmeric
- 1 tsp ground coriander
- 1 red chilli, deseeded and sliced
- 1 large red pepper, diced
- 50g freekeh
- 350ml vegetable stock
- 25g sultanas
- ½ pack coriander, chopped
- 40g cashew nuts

FOR THE RAITA
- 1 garlic clove
- 150ml pot bio-yogurt
- ¼ cucumber, grated
- 2 tbsp chopped mint

1 Chop the garlic for the pilau and set aside. Finely grate the garlic for the raita and put in a bowl. Heat the oil for the pilau in a large open pan, and fry the onion and ginger for 5 mins until softened. Stir in the whole and ground spices, and cook for a few secs to release their aromas. Add the chilli, red pepper and freekeh, stir briefly, then tip in the stock and sultanas. Simmer for 15 mins until the freekeh is tender but still nutty, adding the chopped garlic for the final 2 mins. The stock should have reduced and absorbed into the freekeh now.

2 Meanwhile, finish the raita by stirring the yogurt, cucumber and mint into the grated garlic. When the pilau is cooked, stir in the coriander and cashews, and serve with the cucumber raita.

· ·

GOOD TO KNOW: Vegetarian
PER SERVING kcal 471, fat 20g, saturates 4g, carbs 53g, sugars 27g, fibre 7g, protein 17g, salt 0.2g

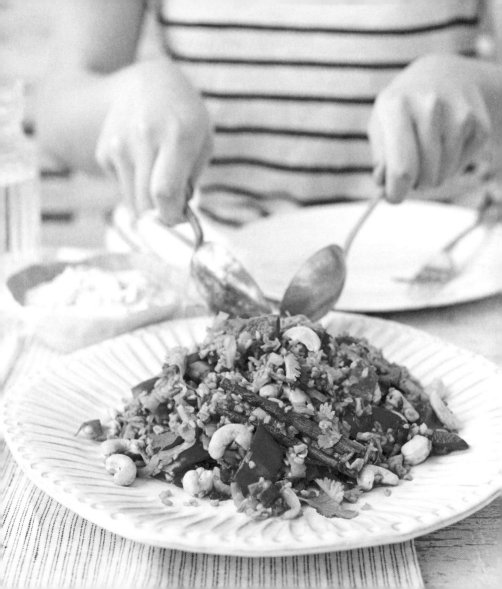

Jerk sweet potato & black bean curry

. . . .

This is a great make-ahead dish, and will last in the fridge for up to 2 days, then all you have to do is finish cooking it on the hob and prepare some rice to serve.

🕐 PREP 50 mins COOK 45 mins 🥧 10

- 2 onions, 1 diced, 1 roughly chopped
- 2 tbsp sunflower oil
- 50g piece ginger, roughly chopped
- small bunch coriander, leaves and stalks separated
- 3 tbsp jerk seasoning
- 2 thyme sprigs
- 400g can chopped tomatoes
- 4 tbsp red wine vinegar
- 3 tbsp demerara sugar
- 2 vegetable stock cubes, crumbled
- 1kg sweet potatoes, peeled and cut into chunks
- 2 x 400g cans black beans, rinsed and drained
- 450g jar roasted red pepper, cut into thick slices

1 Gently soften the diced onion in the sunflower oil in a big pan or casserole.

2 Meanwhile, whizz together the roughly chopped onion, ginger, coriander stalks and jerk seasoning with a blender. Add to the softened onion and fry until fragrant. Stir in the thyme, chopped tomatoes, vinegar, sugar and stock cubes with 600ml water and bring to a simmer. Simmer for 10 mins, then drop in the sweet potatoes and simmer for 10 mins more. Stir in the beans, peppers and some seasoning, and simmer for another 5-10 mins until the potatoes are almost tender. Cool and chill for up to 2 days.

3 To serve, gently heat through on the hob. Roughly chop most of the coriander leaves and stir in, then serve scattered with the remaining leaves.

. . . .
GOOD TO KNOW: Vegan
PER SERVING kcal 209, fat 3g, saturates 1g, carbs 39g, sugars 14g, fibre 7g, protein 6g, salt 0.7g,

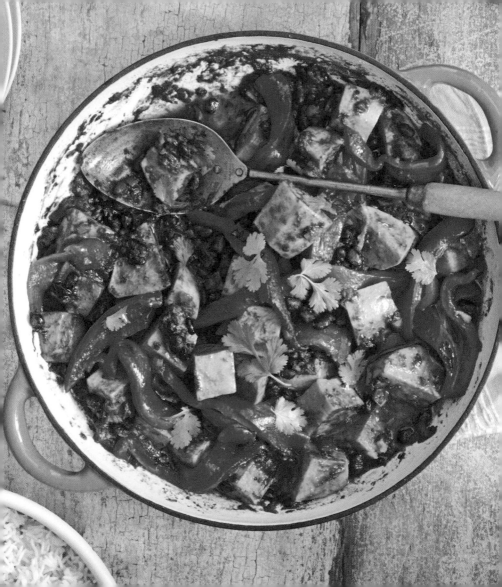

Vietnamese veggie hotpot

Fresh ginger adds spicy warmth without being too fiery.

PREP 5 mins COOK 20 mins | 4

- 2 tsp vegetable oil
- thumb-size piece ginger, shredded
- 2 garlic cloves, chopped
- ½ large butternut squash, peeled and cut into chunks
- 2 tsp soy sauce
- 2 tsp soft brown sugar
- 200ml vegetable stock
- 100g green beans, trimmed and sliced
- 4 spring onions, sliced
- coriander leaves, to serve
- cooked basmati or jasmine rice, to serve

1 Heat the oil in a medium-sized lidded saucepan. Add the ginger and garlic, then stir-fry for about 5 mins. Add the squash, soy sauce, sugar and stock. Cover, then simmer for 10 mins.

2 Remove the lid, add the green beans, then cook for 3 mins more until the squash and beans are tender. Stir the spring onions through at the last minute, then sprinkle with coriander and serve with rice.

GOOD TO KNOW: Vegan
PER SERVING kcal 75, fat 2g, saturates 0g, carbs 13g, sugars 9g, fibre 0g, protein 2g, salt 0.53g

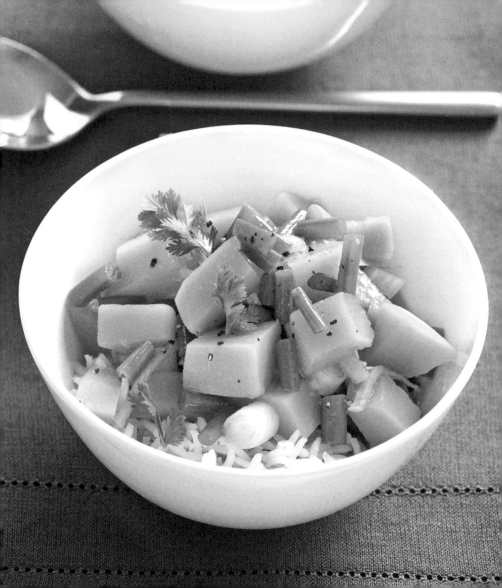

Spiced okra curry

· · · · · · · · · · · · · · · · · · · ·

Simple, delicious and ready in under an hour – ideal for a weeknight supper.

🕐 PREP 15 mins COOK 40 mins 🍽 4

- 5 tbsp olive oil
- 400g onions, sliced
- 500g okra, trimmed, washed, dried and sliced into 2cm pieces
- 2 tomatoes, diced
- 1 red chilli, finely chopped (or ½ tsp powdered)
- 2 tsp ground coriander
- handful coriander, roughly chopped, to serve

1 Heat a large wok or frying pan over a medium heat. Add the oil, then the onions, cooking until soft. Stir in the okra. Add the tomatoes and chilli, then season. Mix well and keep stirring gently, taking care not to break up the okra. Okra releases a sticky substance when cooked, but keep cooking, stirring gently – this will disappear and the tomatoes will become pulpy, about 10 mins.

2 Lower the heat, add the ground coriander and cook for another 5-10 mins. Add 2 tbsp water, cover and let simmer for another 4-5 mins. Sprinkle with coriander and serve with basmati rice or chapati bread.

· ·
GOOD TO KNOW: Vegan
PER SERVING kcal 209, fat 16g, saturates 2g, carbs 13g, sugars 10g, fibre 6g, protein 5g, salt 0.04g

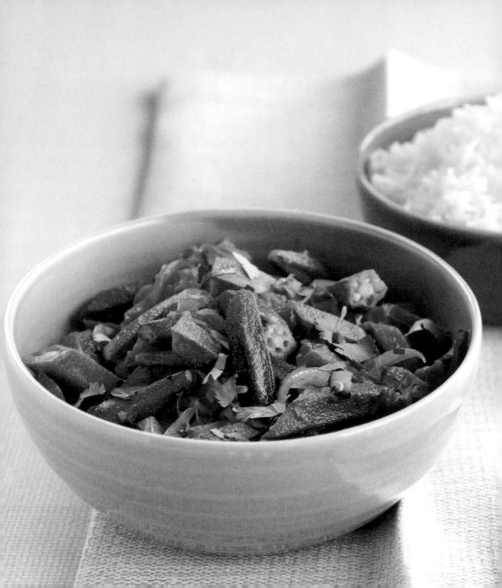

Lentil ragu with courgetti

A satisfying supper that includes a whopping five of your five-a-day.

🕐 PREP 15 mins COOK 40 mins 🥧 4-6

- 2 tbsp extra virgin rapeseed oil, plus 1 tsp
- 3 celery sticks, chopped
- 2 carrots, chopped
- 4 garlic cloves, chopped
- 2 onions, finely chopped
- 140g button mushrooms from a 280g pack, quartered
- 500g pack dried red lentils
- 500g carton passata
- 1 litre reduced-salt vegetable bouillon (we used Marigold)
- 1 tsp dried oregano
- 2 tbsp balsamic vinegar
- 1-2 large courgettes, cut into noodles with a spiraliser, julienne peeler or knife

1 Heat the 2 tbsp oil in a large sauté pan. Add the celery, carrots, garlic and onions, and fry for 4-5 mins over a high heat to soften and start to colour. Add the mushrooms and fry for 2 mins more.

2 Stir in the lentils, passata, bouillon, oregano and balsamic vinegar. Cover the pan and leave to simmer for 30 mins until the lentils are tender and pulpy. Check occasionally and stir to make sure the mixture isn't sticking to the bottom of the pan; if it does, add a drop of water.

3 To serve, heat the remaining oil in a separate frying pan, add the courgette and stir-fry briefly to soften and warm through. Serve half the ragu with the courgetti and chill the rest to eat on another day. Can be frozen for up to 3 months.

GOOD TO KNOW: Vegan
PER SERVING kcal 578, fat 7g, saturates 1g, carbs 87g, sugars 19g, fibre 14g, protein 35g, salt 0.2g

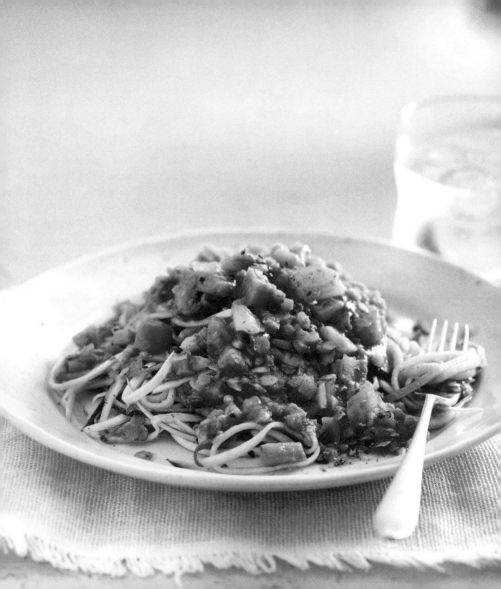

Veggie chilli

This chilli recipe is ready in a flash and couldn't be easier to put together.

🕐 PREP 2 mins COOK 30 mins 🥧 2

- 400g pack oven-roasted vegetables
- 1 can kidney beans in chilli sauce
- 1 can chopped tomatoes
- 1 ready-to-eat mixed grain pouch

1 Heat oven to 200C/180C fan/ gas 6. Cook the vegetables in a casserole dish for 15 mins. Tip in the beans and tomatoes, season, and cook for another 10-15 mins until piping hot. Heat the mixed grain pouch in the microwave on High for 1 min and serve with the chilli.

GOOD TO KNOW: Vegan
PER SERVING kcal 608, fat 14g, saturates 2g, carbs 88g, sugars 30g, fibre 21g, protein 22g, salt 2.4g

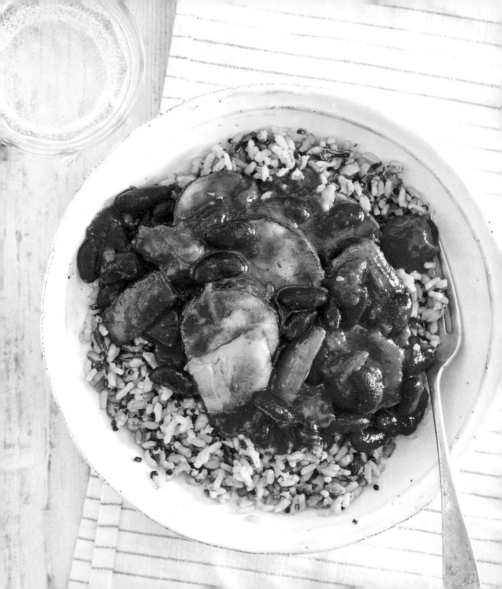

Chard, sweet potato & peanut stew

You don't have to use chard - use any leafy greens you like in this stew, so it's great for using up a glut.

🕐 PREP 15 mins COOK 45 mins 🥧 4

- 2 tbsp sunflower oil
- 1 large onion, chopped
- 1 tsp cumin seeds
- 400g sweet potatoes, cut into medium chunks
- ½ tsp chilli flakes
- 400g can chopped tomato
- 140g salted, roasted peanuts
- 250g chard, leaves and stems, washed and roughly chopped

1 Heat a large saucepan with a lid over a medium heat and add the oil. Add the onion and fry until light golden. Stir in the cumin seeds until fragrant, about 1 min, then add the sweet potato, chilli flakes, tomatoes and 750ml water. Stir, cover and bring to the boil, then uncover and simmer for 15 mins.

2 Meanwhile, whizz the peanuts in a food processor until finely ground, but stop before you end up with peanut butter. Add them to the stew, stir and taste for seasoning – you may want to add a pinch more salt. Simmer for a further 15 mins, stirring frequently.

3 Finally, stir in the chopped chard. Return to the boil and simmer, covered, stirring occasionally, for 8-10 mins or until the chard is cooked. Serve piping hot with plenty of freshly ground black pepper.

GOOD TO KNOW: Vegan
PER SERVING kcal 398, fat 25g, saturates 4g, carbs 33g, sugars 12g, fibre 6g, protein 13g, salt 0.93g

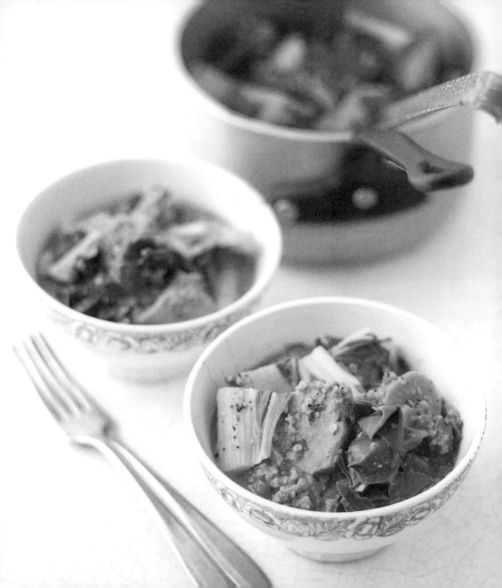

Vegetable vegan biriyani with carrot salad

. . . .

A great sharing dish for a relaxed dinner with friends.

PREP 30 mins plus soaking COOK 40 mins | 8

- 400g basmati rice
- pinch saffron threads (optional)
- 2 tbsp vegetable oil
- 1 cauliflower, cut into florets
- 2 potatoes, cut into chunks
- 100g red lentils
- 100g French beans, trimmed and halved
- handful curry leaves
- 2 handfuls frozen peas
- small bunch coriander
- 50g roasted cashew nuts, roughly chopped

FOR THE PASTE

- 1 large onion, roughly chopped
- large piece ginger, chopped
- 5 garlic cloves
- 2 tsp curry powder
- 1 tsp ground cumin
- 2 tbsp vegetable oil
- 1 small green chilli

1 Soak the rice in cold water for 30 mins, then rinse under running water until the water runs clear. Cover with about 1cm water, add the saffron, cover and bring to the boil, Turn off the heat and stir, then stir again after 10 mins, keeping covered.

2 Blitz the paste ingredients in a food processor. Heat the oil in a saucepan, add the paste, cauliflower and potatoes. Cook in the paste to colour, then add the lentils, green beans, 400ml water and the curry leaves and season. Cover and simmer for 20 mins until the lentils and vegetables are tender. Add the peas for the last 2 mins to defrost. Stir the rice through the curry until completely mixed and hot, then spoon onto a platter and scatter with coriander and cashews.

3 Make a little salad to go alongside. Carrots cut into ribbons and dressed with sugar, lemon juice and mixed nuts and seeds works very well. Serve your salad with the biriyani.

. . . .

GOOD TO KNOW: Vegan
PER SERVING kcal 387, fat 10g, saturates 1g, carbs 59g, sugars 5g, fibre 6g, protein 12g, salt 0.2g

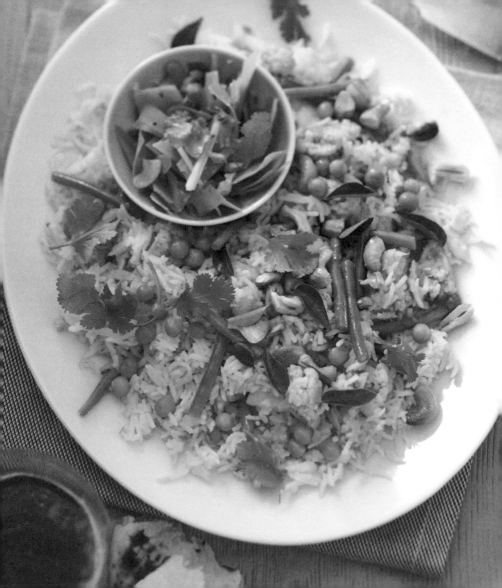

Spiced aubergine bake

Serve comforting bowls of this dish with some fresh crusty bread.

PREP 15 mins COOK 55 mins 4-6

- 4 aubergines, cut into 5mm-1cm slices
- 3 tbsp vegetable oil
- 2 tbsp coconut oil
- 2 large onions, chopped
- 3 garlic cloves, crushed
- 1 tbsp black mustard seeds
- ½ tbsp fenugreek seeds
- 1 tbsp garam masala
- ¼ tsp hot chilli powder
- 1 cinnamon stick
- 1 tsp ground cumin
- 1 tsp ground coriander
- 2 x 400g cans chopped tomatoes
- 200ml coconut milk
- sugar, to taste
- 2 tbsp flaked almonds
- small bunch coriander, roughly chopped (optional)

1 Heat oven to 220C/200C fan/gas 7. Brush each aubergine slice with vegetable oil and place in a single layer on a baking tray or two. Cook on the low shelves for 20 mins, turning once, until golden. Reduce the oven to 180C/160C fan/gas 4.

2 Heat the coconut oil in a large frying pan, add the onions, cover and sweat on a low heat for about 5 mins. Add the garlic, mustard seeds, fenugreek seeds, garam masala, chilli powder, cinnamon stick, cumin and ground coriander. Cook for a few secs until aromatic. Pour in the chopped tomatoes and coconut milk, stir well and season.

3 Spoon a third of the tomato sauce on the bottom of a 2-litre ovenproof dish. Layer with half the aubergine slices. Spoon over a further third of tomato sauce, then the remaining aubergine slices, and finish with the rest of the sauce. Sprinkle over the flaked almonds and coriander (if using), reserving some to serve, and bake for 25-30 mins. Serve garnished with more coriander.

GOOD TO KNOW: Vegan
PER SERVING kcal 318, fat 20g, saturates 9g, carbs 19g, sugars 15g, fibre 12g, protein 8g, salt 0.2g

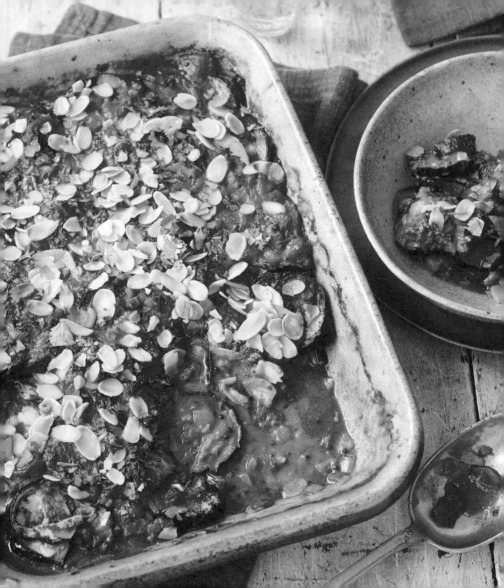

Slow-roast tomato Tatin

To make this vegan use a dairy-free alternative to butter (try sunflower spread) and choose a butter-free puff pastry.

PREP 20 mins COOK 50 mins | 6

- 25g butter or dairy-free alternative
- splash of good olive oil
- 800g medium and small mixed tomatoes, halved across the middle and seeds roughly scooped out
- 1 tbsp light soft brown sugar
- 1 tbsp red wine vinegar
- 1 tbsp thyme leaves or oregano, plus extra to serve
- 375g block puff pastry
- plain flour, for dusting

1 Heat oven to 220C/200C fan/gas 7. Melt the butter with the oil in a wide frying pan. Add the tomatoes, skin-side down, in a single layer (you can do this in batches) and cook over a low heat until they release their juices. Lift out with a slotted spoon into a tart tin (roughly 23cm), skin-side down, cramming them in as they will shrink a little and you don't want any gaps. Add the sugar and vinegar to the pan and cook until the pan juices are reduced and syrupy. Drizzle over the tomatoes, scatter with the oregano or thyme and season.

2 Roll the pastry out on a lightly floured surface to a good 25-26cm round. Lay on top of the tomatoes, and tuck the edges down. Use a fork to prick holes all over the pastry – this will help the steam to escape.

3 Sit the tart tin on a baking tray and bake for 30 mins or until the pastry is golden brown and crisp. Let cool for 10 mins, then run a knife round the edge to release it. Carefully flip the tart over onto a serving plate and scatter with more herbs to serve.

GOOD TO KNOW: Vegetarian
PER SERVING kcal 307, fat 19g, saturates 9g, carbs 29g, sugars 8g, fibre 2g, protein 5g, salt 0.6g

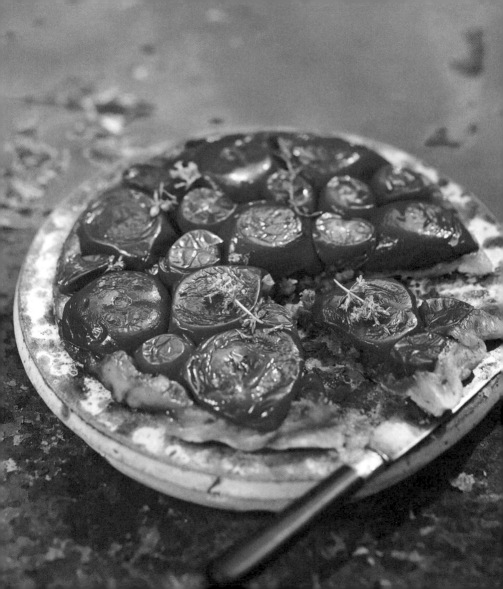

Barley & broccoli risotto with lemon & basil

A low-calorie, satisfying dinner.

PREP 10 mins plus soaking COOK 35 mins 2

- 100g wholegrain pearl barley
- 2 tsp reduced-salt vegetable bouillon powder
- 2 tbsp extra virgin rapeseed oil
- 1 large leek, chopped
- 2 garlic cloves
- ¾ pack basil
- generous squeeze lemon juice
- 125g Tenderstem broccoli from a 200g pack

1 Pour a litre of cold water over the barley, cover and leave to soak overnight.
2 The next day, drain the barley, reserve the liquid and use it to make 500ml vegetable bouillon. Heat half the oil in a non-stick pan, add the leek and cook briefly to soften. Tip half into a bowl, then add the barley and bouillon to the pan, cover and simmer for 20 mins.
3 Meanwhile, add the garlic, basil, remaining oil, the lemon juice and 3 tbsp water to the leeks in the bowl, and blitz to a paste with a stick blender
4 When the barley has cooked for 20 mins, add the broccoli to the pan and cook for 5-10 mins more until both are tender. Stir in the basil purée, heat very briefly (to retain the fragrance), then spoon into bowls to serve.

GOOD TO KNOW: Vegan
PER SERVING kcal 378, fat 14g, saturates 1g, carbs 49g, sugars 5g, fibre 7g, protein 11g, salt 0.1g

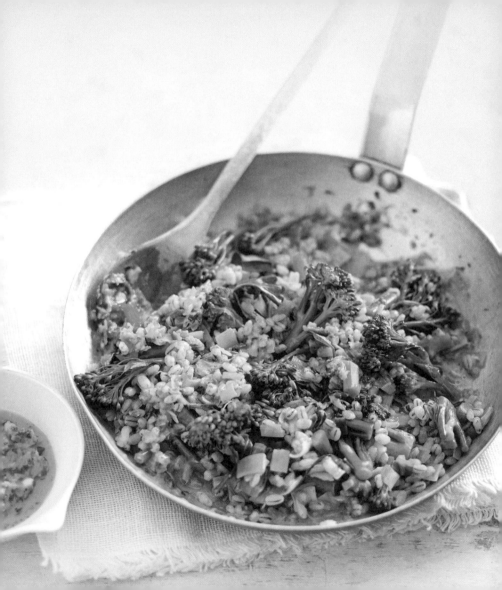

Falafel burgers

Easy to make from storecupboard ingredients.

PREP 10 mins COOK 10 mins 4

- 250g canned chickpeas, drained and rinsed
- 1 medium onion, finely chopped
- 2 garlic cloves, crushed
- 2 tsp ground coriander
- 2 tsp ground cumin
- small pack flat-leaf parsley, chopped
- 2 rounded tbsp plain flour
- 2 tbsp vegetable oil
- 100g houmous
- 4 burger buns, cut in half
- watercress, to serve

1 Dry the chickpeas thoroughly, then tip into the bowl of a food processor. Pulse until lightly broken up into coarse crumbs.

2 Add the onion, garlic, spices, parsley, flour and some seasoning, and continue to pulse until combined. Using your hands, gently form the mixture into 4 patties about 10cm in diameter and 2cm thick.

3 In a large pan, heat the oil and fry the falafels on each side for 2-3 mins or until golden (you may need to do this in batches). Lightly griddle the burger buns on the cut side in a griddle pan, or toast under the grill.

4 Spread one side of each bun with houmous, top with a falafel burger, add a handful of watercress, then pop the remaining bun half on top.

GOOD TO KNOW: Vegan
PER SERVING kcal 476, fat 15g, saturates 2g, carbs 63g, sugars 5g, fibre 7g, protein 17g, salt 2g

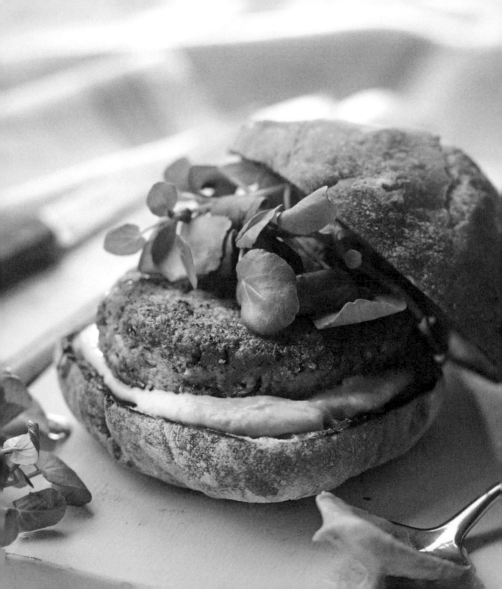

Green masala butternut squash curry

Simple to prepare and big on flavour.

🕐 PREP 10 mins COOK 30 mins 🍴 4

- 40g coriander, plus extra to serve
- 20g mint, stems removed
- 2 green chillies, sliced
- 4 garlic cloves
- 2cm piece ginger, peeled
- 400ml can coconut milk
- 1 tsp garam masala
- 1 tsp ground turmeric
- 500g butternut squash, peeled and cut into even-sized pieces
- 150g green beans, trimmed
- cooked basmati rice, to serve
- mango chutney, to serve

1 Put the herbs, chillies, garlic, ginger and coconut milk in a blender and blend until completely smooth and bright green. (You can use a food processor, but a blender will make a smoother purée because it has 4 blades rather than 2.)

2 Pour the mixture into a medium saucepan and add the spices and 1 tsp salt. Bring to a simmer, add the squash and cook until soft – about 25 mins. Meanwhile, blanch the beans in boiling water, then drain and rinse in cold water – this keeps them perfectly cooked. Add them to the curry just before serving to warm them through. Serve with warm rice, extra coriander and chutney.

GOOD TO KNOW: Vegan
PER SERVING kcal 243, fat 17g, saturates 15g, carbs 15g, sugars 8g, fibre 5g, protein 4g, salt 0.1g

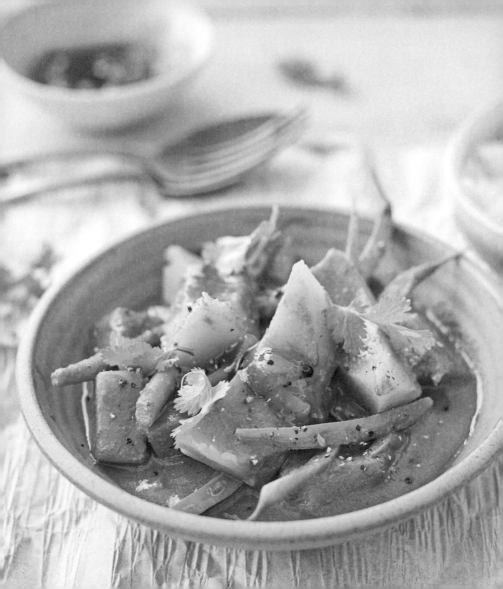

Tofu escalopes with black olive salsa verde

· · · · · · · · · · · · · · · · · · · ·

Use 4 tbsp unsweetened almond milk instead of the egg and combine 50g ground almonds with 2 tbsp nutritional yeast to make a cheese alternative for vegans.

🕐 PREP 20 mins COOK 30 mins 🥧 4

- 600g small new potatoes
- 396g pack firm tofu, drained
- 2 tbsp light soy sauce
- 3 tbsp plain flour
- 50g parmesan-style hard cheese, finely grated
- 2 lemons, both zested, 1 juiced, 1 cut into wedges
- 50g panko or dried breadcrumbs
- 1 egg
- 1 tsp wholegrain mustard
- 2 tbsp vegetable oil, for frying
- 100g bag watercress or rocket

FOR THE SALSA VERDE
- 2 garlic cloves
- 50g basil, stalks chopped
- 2 tbsp small capers
- 4 tbsp extra virgin olive oil, plus extra to serve
- pinch of sugar

1 Boil the potatoes for 20 mins, drain and halve. Cut the well-drained tofu into 8 slices. Lay them on a plate and sprinkle over the soy sauce. Set aside for 5 mins.

2 For the salsa verde, put the garlic, basil, capers, oil and sugar into a food processor with 3 tbsp lemon juice. Pulse until chopped. Stir in the olives and season.

3 Put the flour on a plate and season with pepper. On another plate, combine the cheese, lemon zest and breadcrumbs. Beat the egg, mustard and 2 tsp water in a third bowl. Coat each slice of tofu in the flour, then the egg followed by the breadcrumbs.

4 Heat the vegetable oil in a frying pan over a medium heat. Fry the tofu until golden, about 5 mins each side. Slice into strips and serve with the watercress and potatoes. Spoon over the salsa verde, drizzle over a little extra olive oil and serve with lemon wedges on the side.

· ·

GOOD TO KNOW: Vegetarian
PER SERVING kcal 575, fat 31g, saturates 7g, carbs 50g, sugars 4g, fibre 5g, protein 22g, salt 3.1g

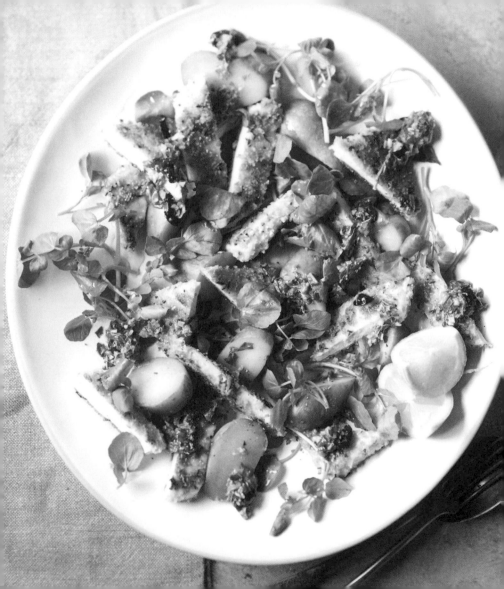

Yaki udon

· ·

Thick and filling wheat noodles work beautifully with earthy mushrooms.

🕐 PREP 10 mins COOK 15 mins 🥧 2

- 250g dried udon noodles (400g frozen or fresh)
- 2 tbsp sesame oil
- 1 onion, thickly sliced
- ¼ head white cabbage, roughly sliced
- 10 shiitake mushrooms
- 4 spring onions, finely sliced

FOR THE SAUCE
- 4 tbsp mirin
- 2 tbsp soy sauce
- 1 tbsp caster sugar
- 1 tbsp Worcestershire sauce (or vegetarian alternative)

1 Boil some water in a large saucepan. Add 250ml cold water and the udon noodles. (As they are so thick, adding cold water helps them to cook a little bit slower so the middle cooks through). If using frozen or fresh noodles, cook for 2 mins or until al dente; dried will take longer, about 5-6 mins. Drain and leave in the colander.

2 Heat 1 tbsp of the oil, add the onion and cabbage and sauté for 5 mins until softened. Add the mushrooms and some spring onions, and sauté for 1 more min. Pour in the remaining sesame oil and the noodles. If using cold noodles, let them heat through before adding to the ingredients for the sauce – otherwise tip in straight away and keep stir-frying until sticky and piping hot. Sprinkle with the remaining spring onions.

· · · · · · · · · · · · · · · · · · · ·
GOOD TO KNOW: Vegetarian
PER SERVING kcal 486, fat 14g, saturates 2g, carbs 73g, sugars 35g, fibre 10g, protein 12g, salt 3.3g

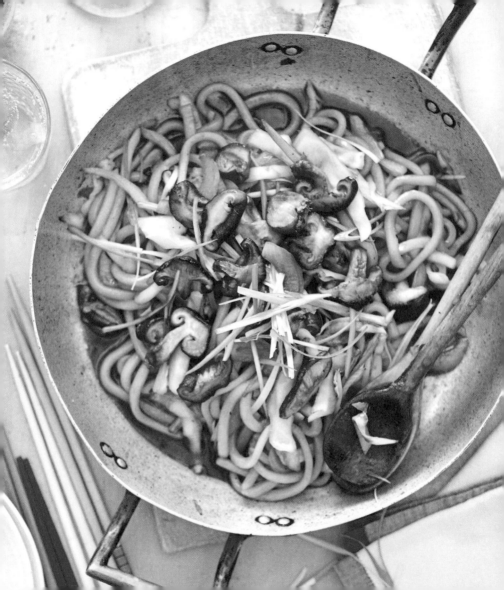

Kadala curry

Serve with rice, dahl and poppadums for a Friday night feast.

⏱ PREP 15 mins COOK 25 mins 🍽 4

FOR THE PASTE
- 2 tbsp oil
- 1 onion, diced
- 1 tsp fresh or dried chilli, to taste
- 9 garlic cloves (approx 1 small bulb of garlic)
- thumb-sized piece ginger, peeled
- 1 tbsp ground coriander
- 2 tbsp ground cumin
- 1 tbsp garam masala
- 2 tbsp tomato purée

FOR THE CURRY
- 2 x 400g cans chickpeas, drained
- 400g can chopped tomatoes
- 100g creamed coconut
- ½ small pack coriander, chopped, plus extra to garnish
- 100g spinach

TO SERVE
- cooked rice and/or dahl

1 To make the paste, heat a little of the oil in a frying pan, add the onion and chilli, and cook until softened, about 8 mins. Meanwhile, in a food processor, roughly combine the garlic, ginger and remaining oil, then add the spices, tomato purée, ½ tsp salt and the fried onion. Blend to a smooth paste – add a drop of water or more oil, if needed.

2 Cook the paste in a saucepan for 2 mins over a medium-high heat, stirring occasionally so it doesn't stick. Tip in the chickpeas and chopped tomatoes and simmer for 5 mins until reduced down. Add the coconut with a little water, cook for 5 mins more, then add the coriander and spinach and cook until wilted. Garnish with extra coriander and serve with rice or dahl (or both).

GOOD TO KNOW: Vegan
PER SERVING kcal 458, fat 28g, saturates 16g, carbs 31g, sugars 9g, fibre 10g, protein 15g, salt 0.2g

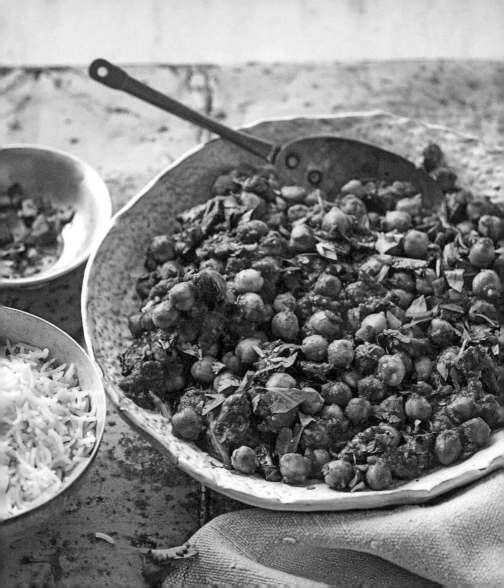

Indian bread with courgettes & coriander

· ·

Also known as thepla, these are best served hot with plain yogurt, or cold with some mango chutney.

PREP 25 mins COOK 50 mins   MAKES 12

- 450g courgettes, grated
- ½ tsp cumin seeds, lightly toasted
- 175g plain flour, plus extra for rolling out
- 175g plain wholemeal flour (not strong bread flour)
- 2 tsp grated ginger
- a good pinch turmeric
- a small handful coriander, chopped
- 3-4 tbsp sunflower oil

1 Tip the courgettes, cumin seeds, both the flours, the ginger, turmeric and coriander into a bowl, add 1 tsp salt and stir well.
2 Pour 1½ tbsp of the oil into the flour mixture and rub it in, then gradually add 4-5 tbsp cold water until the mixture forms a soft dough. Shape into 12 equal-sized balls.
3 Dust the work surface and rolling pin with flour and roll each piece into a thin 14cm round – don't worry if the edges are crinkly.
4 Heat a large frying pan until very hot. Put 1 or 2 breads in the pan and cook for 2 mins each side, patting the edges with a clean soft cloth.
5 Drizzle a little oil around the edges on both sides, then set aside on a plate. Repeat with the rest of the rounds. Serve hot or cold.

· ·
GOOD TO KNOW: Vegan
PER SERVING kcal 257, fat 7g, saturates 1g, carbs 43g, sugars 0g, fibre 4g, protein 8g, salt 0.01g

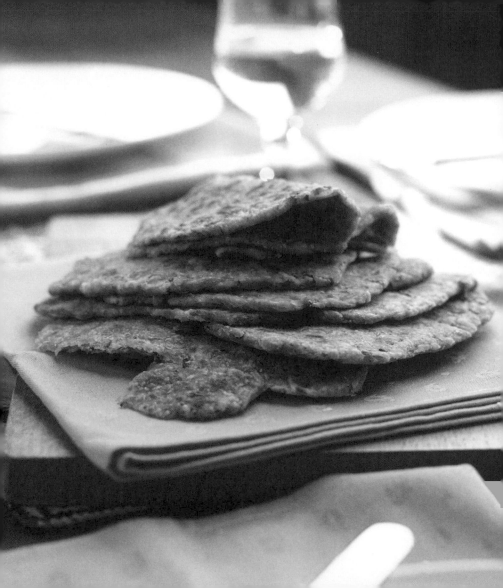

Flowerpot bread

Clay flowerpots need to be treated to stop the bread from sticking. To do this, brush the pots with oil, bake at 200C/180C fan/gas 6 for 1 hr, wash in hot soapy water, then dry.

🕐 PREP 25 mins plus rising COOK 25 mins   🍰 MAKES 5

- 500g granary, strong, wholemeal or white bread flour
- 7g sachet fast-action dried yeast
- 2 tbsp olive oil, plus extra for the flowerpots
- 1 tbsp clear honey
- a little milk or oil, for brushing

PLUS ANY OF THESE TOPPINGS
- 1 tbsp pumpkin, sunflower, sesame or poppy seeds
- 1 tbsp chopped rosemary, thyme, oregano, chives or basil
- 1 tbsp chopped olives or sundried tomatoes
- ½ tsp chilli flakes

YOU WILL ALSO NEED
- 5 small, clean clay flowerpots (see intro above)

1 Tip the flour, yeast and 1 tsp salt into a large bowl. Pour in 300ml warm water, the olive oil and honey. Mix with a wooden spoon until the mixture clumps together, then tip out onto a work surface. Use your hands to stretch and knead the dough for about 10 mins, or until it's smooth and springy. Add a little extra flour if the dough feels too sticky.

2 Brush the flowerpots with oil and line the sides with baking parchment. Divide the dough into 5 pieces and shape into smooth balls. Place one ball of dough into each flowerpot and cover with cling film. Leave in a warm place for 1 hr to rise.

3 Heat oven to 200C/180C fan/gas 6. When the dough has doubled in size, remove the cling film from the pots and gently brush with a little milk or oil. Sprinkle with your choice of topping. Place the pots on a baking tray in the oven and cook for 20-25 mins until risen and golden. The pots will be very hot, so be careful when removing from the oven. Leave to cool for 10 mins before turning out and eating.

GOOD TO KNOW: Vegetarian
PER SERVING kcal 434, fat 8g, saturates 1g, carbs 74g, sugars 4g, fibre 3g, protein 13g, salt 1g

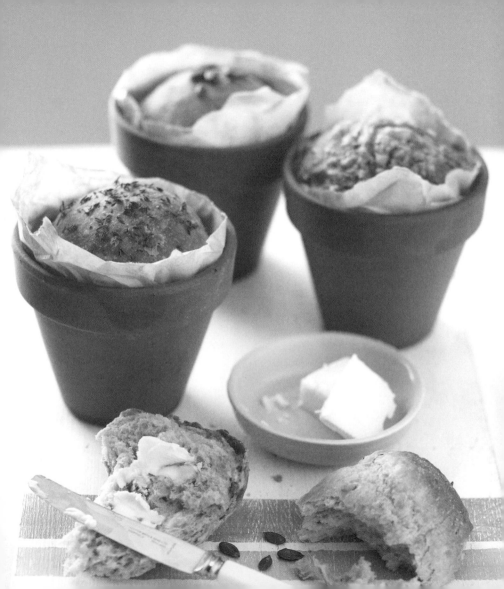

Seeded flatbreads

· ·

These Moroccan-style breads are great for wrapping and dipping.

🕐 PREP 45 mins plus rising COOK 30 mins 🥧 MAKES 12

- 7g sachet fast-action dried yeast
- 1 tsp caster sugar
- 400g strong white bread flour
- 200g wholemeal bread flour
- oil, for greasing
- 1 tbsp black onion seeds
- 2 tbsp sesame seeds

1 Mix the yeast with 2 tbsp warm water and the sugar and leave for a few mins. Tip the flours into a large bowl with 1 tsp salt and make a well in the centre. Pour in the yeast mixture and 500ml warm water. Mix with a wooden spoon until it comes together as a dough, then tip onto a work surface and knead for 5-10 mins until smooth and elastic – add a little extra flour if the dough is too sticky. Put the dough in an oiled bowl, cover with a tea towel and leave in a warm place to rise for 1 hr until doubled in size.

2 Tip the dough onto your work surface and knock out all the air. Knead the seeds into the dough until well distributed. Divide the dough into 12 pieces, then roll out each as thinly as you can. Heat a large frying pan, cook the flatbreads for 2 mins or until bubbles appear on the surface, then flip over and cook for 2 mins more. Once all are cooked, wrap in foil and keep for up to a day. Pop in a warm oven to reheat.

· ·
GOOD TO KNOW: Vegan
PER SERVING kcal 189, fat 3g, saturates 0g, carbs 34g, sugars 1g, fibre 3g, protein 7g, salt 0.4g

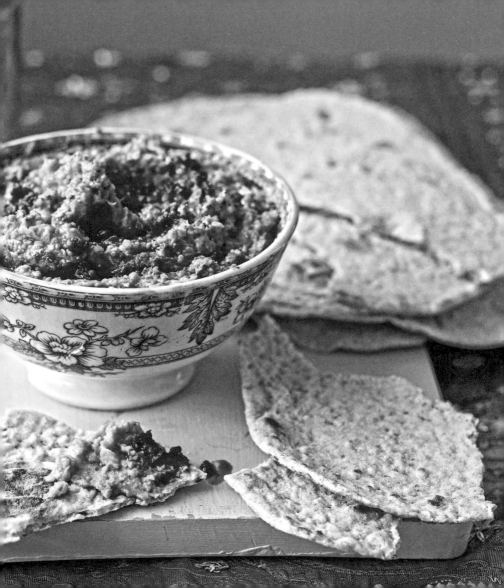

Rye bread

· ·

Use 1 tbsp agave nectar in this recipe if you're avoiding honey.

🕐 PREP 20 mins plus rising COOK 30 mins 📋 MAKES 1 loaf

- 200g rye flour, plus extra for dusting
- 200g strong white or wholemeal flour
- 7g sachet fast-action dried yeast
- ½ tsp fine salt
- 1 tbsp honey
- 1 tsp caraway seeds (optional)

1 Tip the flours, yeast and salt into a bowl. Mix the honey with 250ml warm water, then pour onto the flour and mix to form a soft dough. Add more water if it's too dry. Knead for about 10 mins.

2 Place the dough in a well oiled bowl, cover with cling film and leave to rise in a warm place for 1-2 hrs, or until roughly doubled in size. Dust a 900g loaf tin with flour. Tip the dough back onto your work surface and knead briefly to knock out any air bubbles. If using caraway seeds, work these in to the dough. Shape into a smooth oval loaf and pop into your tin. Cover the tin with oiled cling film and leave to rise somewhere warm for a further 1-1.5 hrs, or until doubled in size.

3 Heat oven to 220C/200C fan/gas 7. Remove the cling film and dust the surface of the loaf with rye flour. Slash a few incisions on an angle then bake for 30 mins until dark brown and hollow sounding when tapped. Transfer to a wire cooling rack and leave to cool for at least 20 mins before serving

· ·

GOOD TO KNOW: Vegetarian
PER SERVING kcal 170, fat 1.1g, saturates 0.2g, carbs 34.3g, sugars 2.3g, fibre 6.9g, protein 5.6g, salt 0.3g

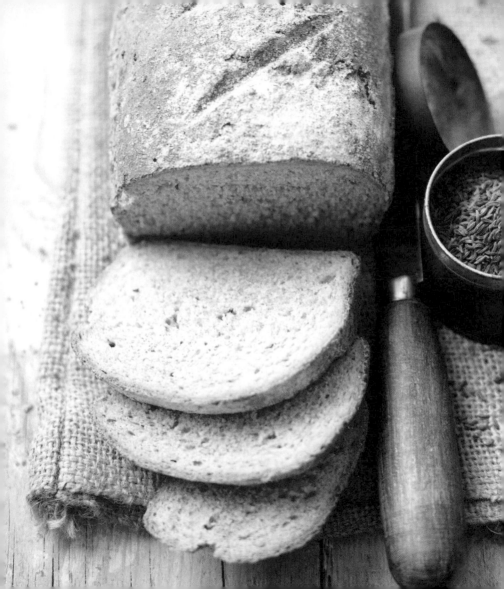

Rainbow rolls

Use up leftover veg to make these savoury scone-style rolls. They're good served warm with nut butter or with soups and stews.

PREP 25 mins plus rising COOK 35 mins   MAKES 18

- 250g plain white flour, plus extra for dusting
- 250g white bread flour
- 500g seed and grain bread flour
- 7g sachet fast-action dried yeast
- 100g porridge oats
- 100g mixed seeds, plus extra for sprinkling
- 50g walnuts, finely chopped
- 2 tsp bicarbonate of soda
- 50g cold sunflower margarine, diced
- 500ml unsweetened almond milk, plus extra to glaze
- 100g grated courgettes
- 100g grated carrots
- 100g grated raw beetroot – wear gloves!

1 Dust your largest baking sheet or tray with flour. Mix the flours, yeast, oats, seeds, nuts, bicarbonate and 2 tsp salt in a bowl, then rub in the margarine with your fingers until it almost disappears.

2 Pour in the almond milk and 150-200ml water and mix quickly with a wooden spoon, then your hands, to form a dough. Divide into 3 and knead a grated veg into each to make a courgette dough, a carrot dough and a beetroot dough. Form each into 6 rounds with floured hands. Arrange, spaced apart, on the baking tray, cover loosely with oiled cling film, and leave to rise somewhere warm for about 30 mins.

3 Heat oven to 200C/180C fan/gas 6. Brush the tops with almond milk, scatter with extra seeds and bake for 30-35 mins until the bases are pale golden and sound hollow when tapped. Cover with a tea towel and leave to cool a bit – this will keep them soft.

GOOD TO KNOW: Vegan
PER SERVING kcal 298, fat 8g, saturates 1g, carbs 44g, sugars 1g, fibre 4g, protein 9g, salt 0.9g

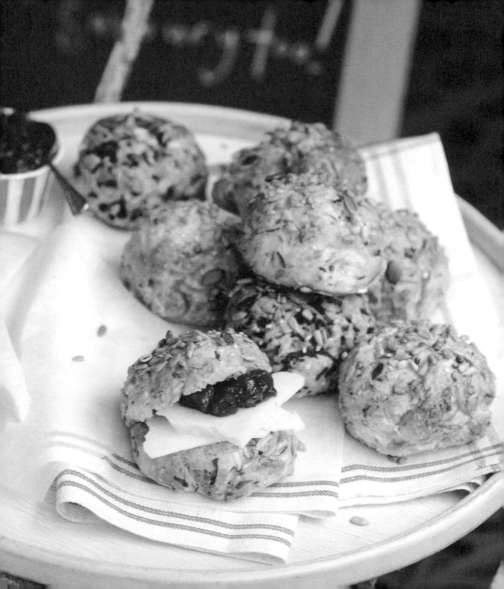

Strawberry & rose sorbet

This refreshing dessert is the ideal end to a spicy meal.

PREP 10 mins plus freezing COOK 5 mins 6

- 300g caster sugar
- 900g ripe strawberries, hulled
- juice 1 lemon
- 2 tbsp rosewater
- handful pink rose petals, to serve (optional)

1 In a medium saucepan, combine the sugar with 300ml water. Let the sugar dissolve, then bring to the boil for 1 min. Put the strawberries in a blender or food processor and pulse until smooth. Trickle in the sugar syrup, blend again, then add the lemon juice and the rosewater.

2 Pour the strawberry mixture into a large freezer-proof container (an old ice cream tub is perfect), then freeze until almost solid, mashing in the ice crystals every 1-2 hrs until the sorbet is thick and smooth. Wrap well and freeze until solid. Allow to soften for 15 mins before scooping and decorating with rose petals, if using. Best eaten within a month.

GOOD TO KNOW: Vegan
PER SERVING kcal 238, fat 0g, saturates 0g, carbs 58g, sugars 58g, fibre 2g, protein 1g, salt 0g

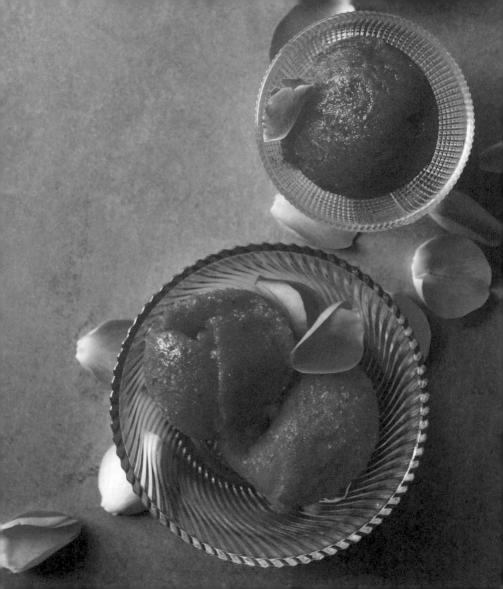

Mango, lime & coconut sundaes

A delicate balance of rich coconut and sharp mango sorbet makes a smart end to a light dinner party menu.

PREP 30 mins plus freezing · 6

- 3 ripe mangoes, peeled, cored and sliced
- juice and zest 2 limes, plus 6 slices
- 500ml tub dairy-free coconut milk ice cream (we used Booja-Booja Coconut Hullabaloo)
- a few mint leaves

1 Put half the mango slices in a bowl with half the lime juice and half the zest, cover and chill until serving. Put the rest of the mango in the freezer for 3-4 hrs or until frozen solid.

2 Put the frozen mango in a blender with the rest of the lime juice and zest (saving a few pinches for decoration), blend until smooth, then tip into a container and leave in the freezer until needed.

3 Just before serving, put the chilled mango pieces in the bottom of 6 sundae glasses and take the coconut ice cream and frozen mango sorbet out of the freezer to defrost just enough to scoop. Divide the mango sorbet and the coconut ice cream among the glasses, and decorate with mint leaves, lime slices and any remaining lime zest.

GOOD TO KNOW: Vegan
PER SERVING kcal 288, fat 10g, saturates 4g, carbs 44g, sugars 40g, fibre 3g, protein 4g, salt 0.1g

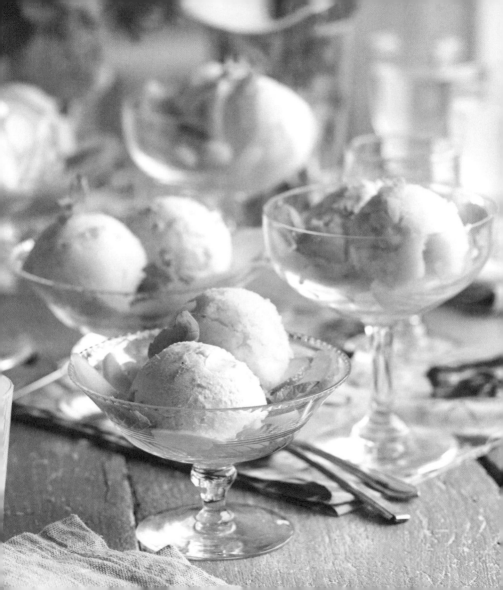

Cherries in rosé wine & vanilla syrup

This light, fresh-tasting dessert looks elegant served in individual glasses. Top it with a spoonful of whipped coconut cream for the perfect finish.

🕐 PREP 10 mins COOK 20 mins 🥧 4

- 425ml rosé wine
- 1 vanilla pod, split lengthways
- 100g demerara sugar
- 500g cherrries

1 Tip the wine into a medium pan, then add the vanilla pod to the pan with the sugar. Bring to the boil, then reduce the heat and simmer until the sugar has dissolved.

2 Stone the cherries if you want, or leave them as they are. Add to the pan and cook gently for 6 mins. Remove with a slotted spoon to a bowl. Increase the heat, then boil the liquid for 8-10 mins until slightly syrupy. Pour over the cherries and serve warm or cold in glass bowls or glasses.

GOOD TO KNOW: *Vegan*
PER SERVING kcal 199, fat 0g, saturates 0g, carbs 43g, sugars 43g, fibre 1g, protein 1g, salt 0.02g

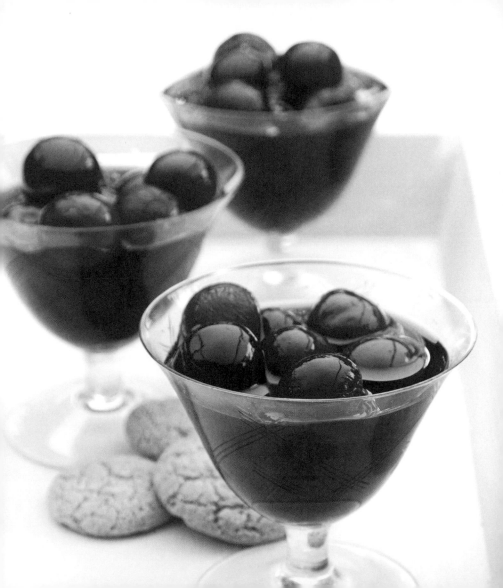

Lemon sorbet

· ·

Serve as a light dessert or as a zingy palate cleanser between courses of a rich menu.

🕐 PREP 10 mins plus freezing COOK 10 mins 🍽 4-6

- 250g white caster sugar
- thick strip lemon peel
- juice 2-3 lemons
- 2 tbsp vodka (optional)

TO SERVE
- zest ½ lemon

1 Heat 250ml water, the sugar and the lemon peel in a small pan until the sugar has dissolved, then bring the mixture to the boil. Cook for 3 mins, then turn off the heat and leave to cool. Pick out the lemon peel and discard. Measure out 100ml of lemon juice and add to the sugar mixture along with the vodka, if using.

2 Pour into a freezer-proof container and freeze for 1 hr 30 mins, then mix up with a whisk to break up and incorporate the ice crystals (which will be starting to form at the edges) before returning to the freezer.

3 Keep mixing the sorbet once an hour for 4 hours to break up the ice crystals. Stop mixing when firm but still scoopable, then store in the freezer for up to 1 month. Serve scoops of sorbet decorated with a few curls of lemon zest.

· ·
GOOD TO KNOW: Vegan
PER SERVING kcal 179, fat 0g, saturates 0g, carbs 42g, sugars 42g, fibre 0g, protein 0g, salt 0g

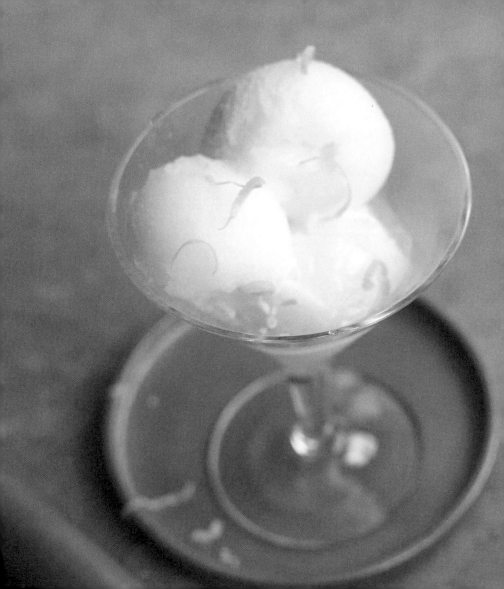

Sticky toffee pear pudding

Just as sticky and buttery as the original but our version is completely vegan.

PREP 25 mins COOK 1 hr 15 mins 8

- 200g golden caster sugar
- 2 cinnamon sticks
- 1 star anise
- 6 cloves
- 1 lemon, zest pared
- 1 orange, zest pared
- 8 small firm pears, peeled and cored through the base
- vegan ice cream, to serve (optional)

FOR THE SPONGE
- 250g pitted dates
- 2 tbsp linseeds
- 300ml unsweetened almond milk
- 200ml vegetable oil, plus extra for greasing
- 175g dark muscovado sugar 200g self-raising flour
- 1 tsp bicarbonate of soda
- 1 tsp ground mixed spice

1 Tip the caster sugar, whole spices, zests and 600ml water into a saucepan and simmer to dissolve the sugar. Add the pears and poach for 15 mins, the leave to cool.

2 Put the dates, linseeds and almond milk in a saucepan. Simmer for 2-3 mins, then blitz in a food processer until smooth.

3 Heat oven to 180C/160C fan/gas 4. Grease and line a 20 x 30cm baking tin.

4 Mix the muscovado sugar, flour, bicarb and mixed spice in a bowl with the oil, date mixture and ½ tsp salt. Pour into the tin and nestle in the pears, standing them upright. Bake for 35-40 mins, then bake for 10 mins more if a skewer doesn't come out cleanly. Bring the poaching liquid back to the boil and simmer until syrupy, then brush all over the cake. Serve with extra syrup and a scoop of vegan ice cream

GOOD TO KNOW: Vegan
PER SERVING kcal 646, fat 27g, saturates 2g, carbs 94g, sugars 75g, fibre 6g, protein 4g, salt 0.9g

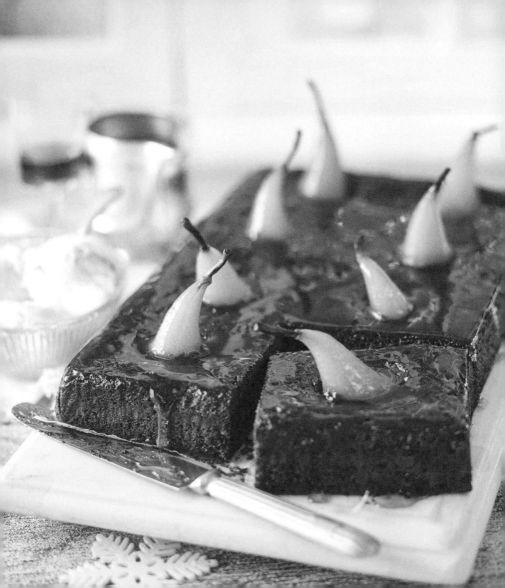

Red berry fruit compote (German rote grütze)

· ·

Choose a dairy-free custard or serve with scoops of vegan ice cream, if you prefer.

🕐 PREP 5 mins plus chilling COOK 25 mins 🍴 6 with leftovers

- 440g canned pitted cherries in syrup (Morello or sour cherries are best, if you can get them)
- 100g mixed fresh or frozen forest fruits (blackberries, blueberries, raspberries, strawberries)
- 180ml cranberry juice
- ½ tbsp vanilla extract
- ½ tsp ground cinnamon
- ½ tbsp golden caster sugar
- dash rosewater
- 2 tbsp cornflour
- 500g pot good-quality vanilla custard

TO DECORATE
- 1 square 70% dark chocolate, finely grated
- handful pomegranate seeds
- handful mint leaves

1 In a large saucepan over a medium heat, cook the fruits in their juices and syrup, along with 150ml of the cranberry juice, the vanilla extract, cinnamon, sugar and rosewater for about 20 mins or until the fruits are soft.

2 In a separate bowl, mix the remaining cranberry juice with the cornflour until it becomes smooth and milky without any lumps. Pour slowly into the hot fruit and continue stirring until mixed in well – the compote will thicken after a couple of mins. Remove from the heat and leave to cool. Transfer to a bowl, cover and chill in the fridge for a few hours before serving for best results in texture and flavour. Will keep for up to 1 week.

3 Serve the compote in ramekins, small bowls or clean jam jars, with a generous dollop of vanilla custard. Sprinkle the chocolate shavings and pomegranate seeds on top, and finish with the mint leaves.

· ·

GOOD TO KNOW: Vegetarian
PER SERVING kcal 171, fat 2g, saturates 2g, carbs 33g, sugars 24g, fibre 1g, protein 3g, salt 0.1g

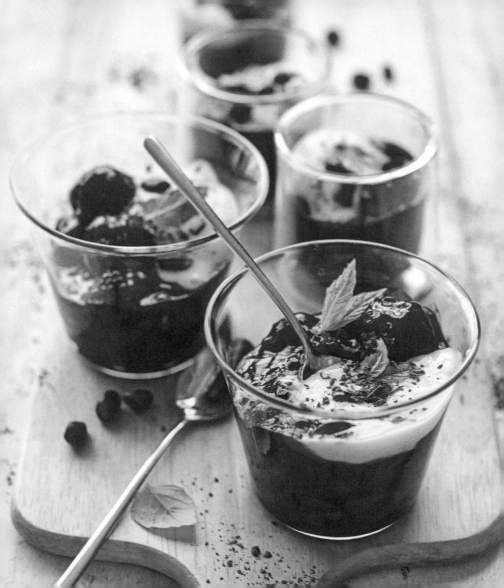

Chai coconut & mango creams

This smart dessert will leave all your guests wowed.

PREP 30 mins plus chilling COOK 20 mins 4

- 2 x 400ml cans full-fat coconut milk
- 4 allspice berries, crushed
- 4 cardamom pods, crushed
- 1 cinnamon stick
- 3 cloves
- 1 vanilla pod, split, or ½ tsp vanilla extract
- 200g caster sugar
- a little vegetable or sunflower oil, for greasing
- 1 ripe mango, 1 cheek cut into small dice and set aside to serve, remaining 140g roughly chopped
- juice ½ lime
- 4 tbsp agar-agar flakes (find in health food shops)
- 2 crinkly passion fruits, to serve
- mint leaves, to serve
- toasted coconut shavings, to serve

1 Simmer the coconut milk, spices, vanilla and 140g of the caster sugar in a pan for 5 mins, then chill overnight.

2 Oil 4 x 200ml ramekins. Purée the remaining sugar, chopped mango and lime juice in a food processor. Sieve into a saucepan, sprinkle 1 tbsp agar-agar flakes over the surface and leave until it dissolves. Stir and bring to a simmer for 3-5 mins until it has thickened slightly. Divide among the moulds and chill for at least 2 hrs.

3 Sieve the coconut milk into a pan to remove the spices. Sprinkle over the remaining agar-agar and leave until dissolved. Simmer and stir for 3-5 mins. Divide among the moulds and chill for 4 hrs.

4 Dip the base of each mould into hot water and turn out onto plates. Top with the diced mango, passion fruit seeds, sprig of mint and coconut flakes.

. . . .

GOOD TO KNOW: Vegan
PER SERVING kcal 626, fat 37g, saturates 30g, carbs 68g, sugars 64g, fibre 4g, protein 3g, salt 0g

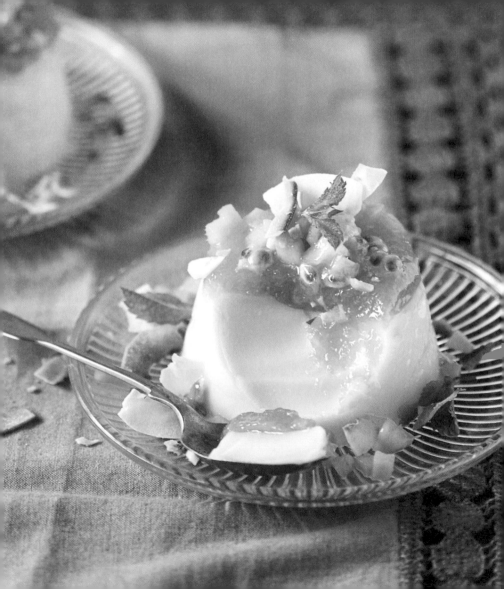

Chocolate banana ice cream

Perfect for when you want a quick and easy chocolatey pud.

🕐 5 mins 🥧 1

- 1 frozen banana
- 1 tsp cocoa powder

In a blender, blitz the frozen banana with the cocoa powder until smooth. Eat straight away.

GOOD TO KNOW: Vegan
PER SERVING kcal 110, fat 1g, saturates 0g, carbs 23g, sugars 21g, fibre 2g, protein 2g, salt 0g

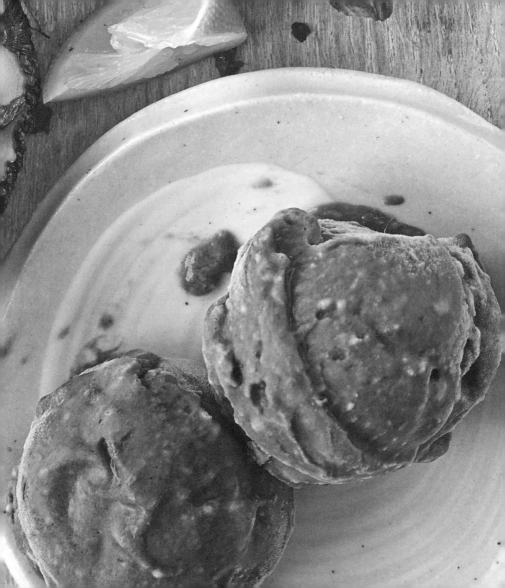

Cheat's pineapple, Thai basil & ginger sorbet

Bursting with tropical flavour.

🕐 PREP 5 mins plus overnight chilling   🥧 6

- 1 large pineapple, peeled, cored and cut into chunks
- juice and zest 1 lime
- 1 small piece ginger, sliced
- handful Thai basil leaves, plus a few extra little ones to serve
- 75g white caster sugar
- vodka or white rum, for drizzling (optional)

1 A couple of days before eating, tip everything into a blender or smoothie maker with 200ml water and blitz until very smooth. Pour into a freezer-proof container and freeze overnight until solid.

2 A few hours before serving, remove from the freezer and allow to defrost slightly so it slides out of the container in a block. Chop the block into ice cube-sized chunks and blitz in the blender or smoothie maker again until you have a thick, slushy purée. Tip back into the container and refreeze for 1 hr or until it can be scooped out.

3 To serve, scoop the sorbet into chilled bowls or glasses and top with extra basil. If you want you can drizzle with something a little more potent, such as vodka or white rum.

GOOD TO KNOW: Vegan
PER SERVING kcal 145, fat 0g, saturates 0g, carbs 33g, sugars 33g, fibre 3g, protein 1g, salt 0g

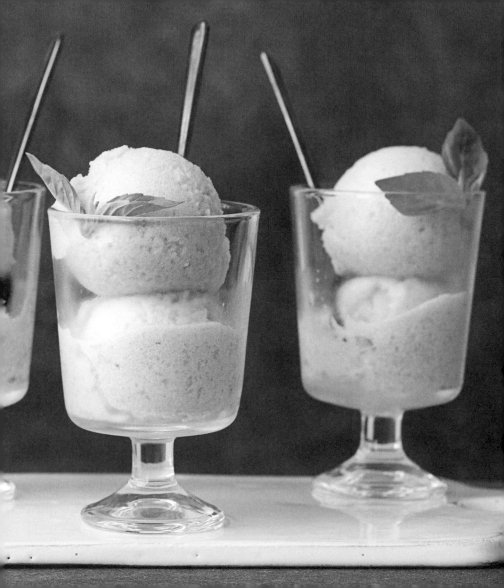

Blueberry & coconut frozen 'cheesecake' bars

Make a batch of these and keep them in the freezer for a handy, delicious vegan dessert anytime.

PREP 25 mins plus soaking and freezing   MAKES 10-12

- 280g unsalted cashew nuts, soaked overnight and drained
- flavourless oil, for greasing

FOR THE BASE
- 140g unsalted almonds
- 140g pitted dates

FOR THE 'CHEESECAKE' LAYER
- 100g coconut cream
- 2 tbsp coconut oil, melted
- 2 tbsp clear honey
- 1 tsp vanilla extract
- juice ½ lemon

FOR THE TOPPING
- 140g blueberries, plus a handful
- 5 pitted dates

1 Oil a 20 x 20cm square cake tin. Make the base by whizzing the almonds and dates in a food processor until finely chopped. Tip into your prepared tin and press down with the back of a spoon. Put the tin in the freezer to firm up.

2 Put half the cashews in the food processor. Add the 'cheesecake' layer ingredients and blitz until creamy. Spread on top of the base and return to the freezer for 30-40 mins.

3 In a food processor blend the blueberries, dates and remaining cashews. Take the tin out of the freezer and spoon over the topping, then scatter over a handful of whole blueberries. Freeze for 1 hr to firm up. (Keeps in the freezer for up to 2 months.) Remove from the freezer 10 mins before slicing.

GOOD TO KNOW: Vegan
PER SERVING kcal 329, fat 32g, saturates 6g, carbs 24g, sugars 20g, fibre 3g, protein 8g, salt 0g

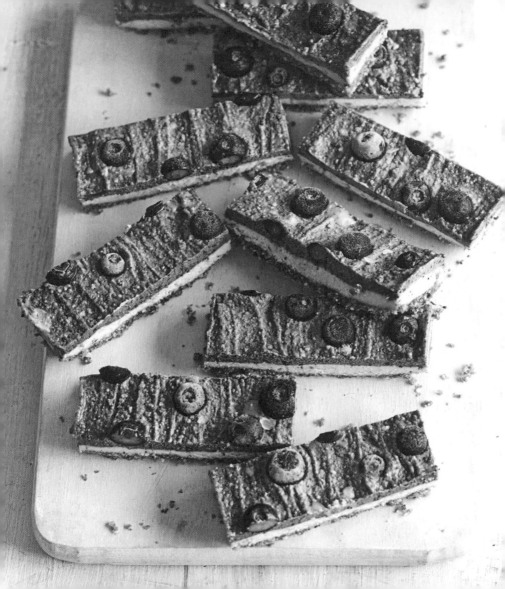

Instant berry banana slush

A healthy, sweet treat you can make in minutes.

🕐 5 mins 🥧 2

- 2 ripe bananas
- 200g frozen berry mix (blackberries, raspberries and currants)

Slice the bananas into a bowl and add the frozen berry mix. Blitz with a stick blender to make a slushy ice and serve straight away in 2 glasses with spoons.

GOOD TO KNOW: Vegan
PER SERVING kcal 119, fat 0.4g, saturates 0.1g, carbs 24g, sugars 22g, fibre 5g, protein 2g, salt 0g

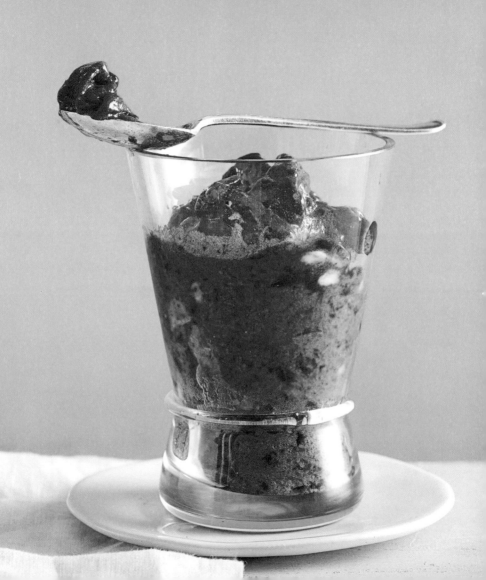

Feelgood flapjacks

Bananas and apples bind the mixture, so you can cut down on the fat and sugar.

PREP 10 mins COOK 1 hr MAKES 12

- 50g butter or dairy-free sunflower spread
- 2 tbsp smooth peanut butter
- 3 tbsp maple syrup
- 2 ripe bananas, mashed
- 1 apple, peeled and grated
- 250g rolled oats
- 85g dried apricots, chopped
- 100g raisins
- 85g mixed seeds (we used pumpkin and sunflower)

1 Heat oven to 160C/140C fan/gas 3. Grease and line a 20cm square tin with baking parchment. Heat the butter, peanut butter and maple syrup in a small pan until melted. Add the mashed banana, apple and 100ml hot water, and mix to combine.

2 Tip the oats, the dried fruit and the seeds into a large bowl. Pour in the combined banana and apple and stir until everything is coated by the wet mixture. Tip into the cake tin and level the surface. Bake for 55 mins or until golden. Leave to cool in the tin. Cut into 12 pieces to serve or store in an airtight container in the fridge. They will keep for up to 3 days.

GOOD TO KNOW: Vegetarian
PER SERVING kcal 218, fat 8g, saturates 3g, carbs 29g, sugars 17g, fibre 4g, protein 6g, salt 0.1g

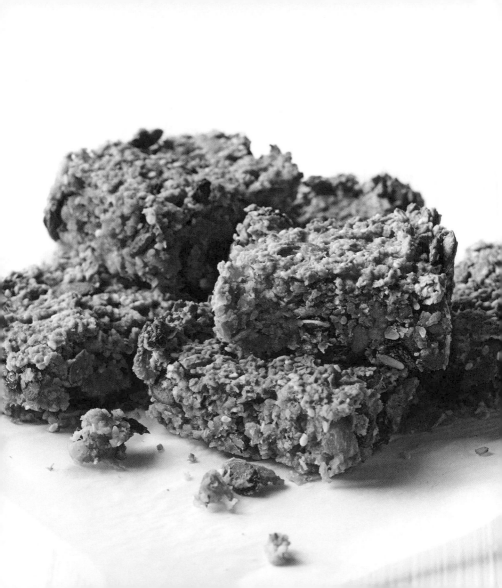

Oaty hazelnut cookies

Soft and slightly chewy, these oaty cookies work equally well made with butter and egg as they do as a vegan version with sunflower spread and chia seeds.

🕐 PREP 15 mins COOK 30 mins 🥧 MAKES 9

- 50g butter or dairy-free sunflower spread
- 2 tbsp maple syrup
- 1 dessert apple, unpeeled and coarsely grated (you need 85g)
- 1 tsp ground cinnamon
- 50g raisins
- 50g porridge oats
- 50g spelt flour
- 40g unblanched hazelnuts, cut into chunky slices
- 1 egg or 1 chia egg (chia egg is 1 tbsp chia seeds soaked for 5 mins in 3 tbsp water until the mixture becomes gloopy)

1 Heat oven to 180C/160C fan/gas 4 and lightly grease a non-stick baking tray (or line a normal baking tray with baking parchment). Tip the butter and syrup into a small non-stick pan and melt together, then add the apple and cook, stirring, over a medium heat until it softens, about 6-7 mins. Stir in the cinnamon and raisins.

2 Mix the oats, spelt flour and hazelnuts in a bowl, pour in the apple mixture, then add the egg and beat everything together really well.

3 Spoon onto the baking tray, well spaced apart to make 9 mounds, then gently press into discs. Bake for 18-20 mins until golden, then cool on a wire rack. Will keep for 3 days in an airtight container or up to 6 weeks in the freezer.

GOOD TO KNOW: Vegetarian
PER SERVING kcal 146, fat 8g, saturates 3g, carbs 15g, sugars 8g, fibre 2g, protein 2g, salt 0.1g

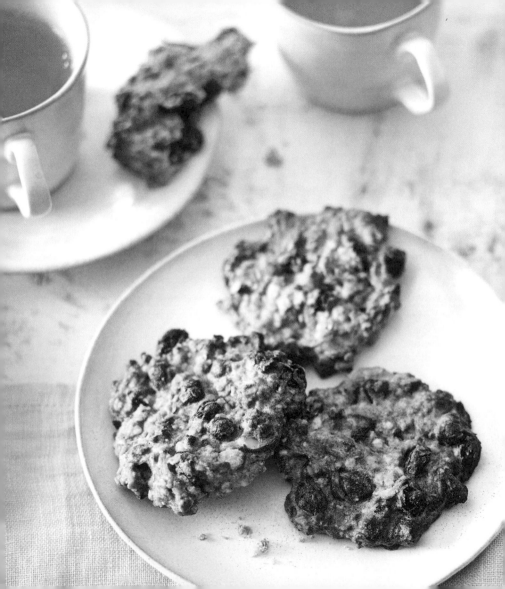

Key lime & coconut pie

A creamy, rich dessert.

PREP 35 mins plus chilling COOK 10 mins   12

FOR THE BASE
- 300g Hobnobs
- 75g coconut oil, melted, plus extra for greasing

FOR THE FILLING
- 200g cashew nuts, soaked overnight and drained
- juice 7 limes, plus zest of 2
- 300g silken tofu
- 150g coconut oil, melted
- 100ml maple syrup

TO SERVE
- zest 1 lime or lime slices
- whipped coconut cream or coconut yogurt (optional)

1 Heat oven to 160C/140C fan/gas 3. Whizz the biscuits to crumbs in a food processor, then tip into a large bowl and stir in the melted coconut oil. Grease a 22cm loose-based fluted tart tin with a little coconut oil, then press the biscuit mixture into the base and up the sides. Bake in the oven for 10 minutes, then remove and leave to cool completely.

2 To prepare the filling, blend all the ingredients in a high-speed blender on a high-speed setting or in a food processor until they are very smooth.

3 Pour the filling into the crust and shake the base gently to level out the mixture. Chill in the fridge overnight or place in the freezer for 25-30 mins before serving or until set. Decorate with the lime zest and whipped coconut cream or lime slices, if you like.

GOOD TO KNOW: *Vegan*
PER SERVING kcal 424, fat 33g, saturates 19g, carbs 24g, sugars 12g, fibre 2g, protein 6g, salt 0.2g

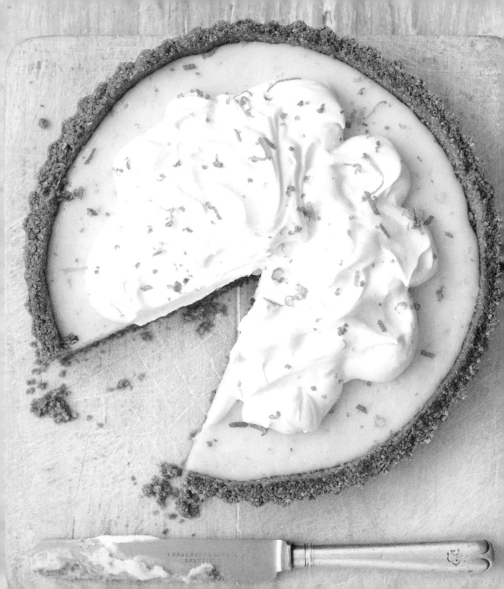

Chocolate avocado cake

· · · · · · · · · · · · · · · · · · · ·

An indulgent, squidgy chocolate cake that you'd never guess is free from dairy, eggs and nuts.

🕐 PREP 30 mins plus cooling COOK 35 mins 🥧 12-16

FOR THE CAKE
- dairy-free sunflower spread, for greasing
- 150g ripe avocado, mashed
- 300g light muscovado sugar
- 350g gluten-free plain flour
- 50g cocoa powder
- 1 tsp bicarbonate of soda
- 2 tsp baking powder
- 400ml unsweetened soya milk
- 150ml vegetable oil
- 2 tsp vanilla extract

FOR THE FROSTING
- 85g avocado, mashed
- 85g dairy-free sunflower spread
- 200g dairy-free chocolate, chopped
- 125ml unsweetened soya milk
- 25g cocoa powder
- 200g icing sugar
- 1 tsp vanilla extract
- vegan sprinkles, to decorate

1 Heat oven to 160C/140C fan/gas 3. Grease and line 2 x 20cm sandwich tins. Blend the avocado and sugar in a food processor until smooth. Add the rest of the cake ingredients plus ½ tsp salt and process until liquid. Divide between the tins and bake for 25 mins or until cooked through. Cool in the tins for 5 mins, then turn out onto wire racks until cold.

2 For the frosting, beat the avocado and sunflower spread with electric beaters until smooth, then sieve. Melt the chocolate in the microwave. Bring the soya milk to a simmer, then gradually sift in the cocoa and mix until smooth. Off the heat add in the avocado mix, icing sugar, melted chocolate and vanilla, and beat until shiny. Use this to sandwich and top the cake. Leave to set for 10 mins before decorating with sprinkles and slicing.

· ·
GOOD TO KNOW: Vegan
PER SERVING kcal 452, fat 24g, saturates 6g, carbs 53g, sugars 34g, fibre 3g, protein 4g, salt 0.9g

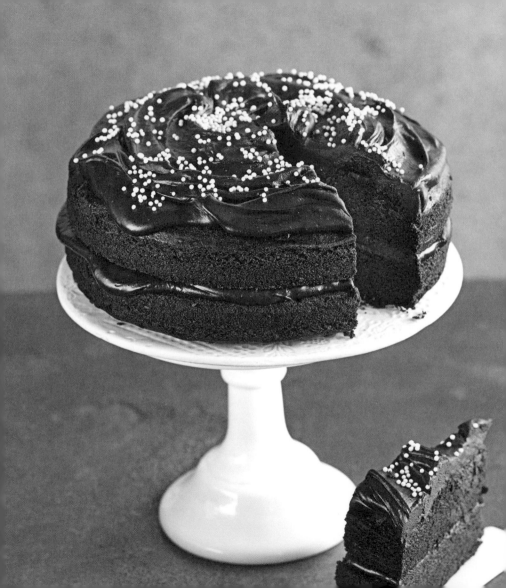

Vegan banana & peanut butter cupcakes

Sure to be a firm favourite with vegans and non-vegans alike.

🕐 PREP 25 mins COOK 20 mins 🕐 MAKES 16

- 240g self-raising flour
- 140g golden caster sugar
- 1 tsp bicarbonate of soda
- 240g egg-free mayonnaise
- 2 large or 3 small ripe bananas, mashed
- 1 tsp vanilla extract
- 25g vegan dark chocolate chips

FOR THE ICING
- 80g vegan margarine
- 250g icing sugar
- 25ml vegan milk (we used almond milk)
- 2 tbsp smooth peanut butter

1 Heat oven to 170C/150C fan/gas 3½. Line muffin tins with 16 paper cases. In a bowl, combine the flour, sugar, ½ tsp salt and the bicarbonate of soda. In a second bowl or a jug, mix the mayonnaise, mashed bananas and vanilla extract. Pour the wet ingredients into the dry and mix with a spoon until just combined (don't overmix or your cupcakes will be heavy). Spoon the mixture into the cases and bake for 20 mins.

2 When the cupcakes come out of the oven, sprinkle the choc chips over – they will melt and then harden again, so don't touch them.

3 For the icing, combine the vegan margarine and icing sugar in an electric mixer, then add the vegan milk and continue to mix on a slow speed until completely combined. Turn the mixer up and combine for a further 3 mins. Finally, stir in the peanut butter. Pipe or simply spread the icing on top of the cakes. Store in an airtight container and eat within 2 days.

GOOD TO KNOW: Vegan
PER SERVING kcal 295, fat 14g, saturates 3g, carbs 40g, sugars 28g, fibre 1g, protein 2g, salt 0.7g

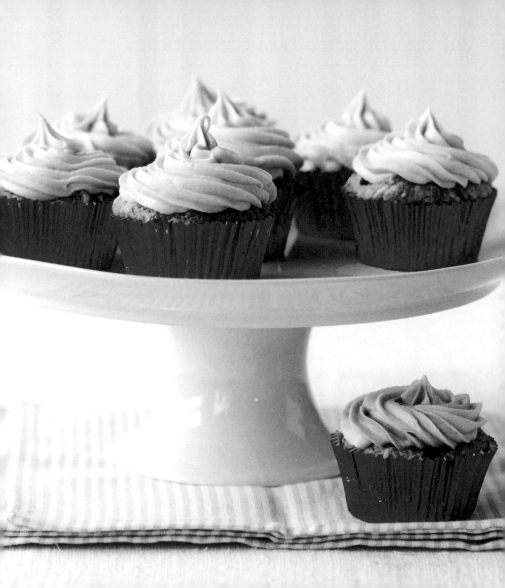

Vegan rhubarb & custard bake

A comforting pudding that's great with extra custard when still warm from the oven or cold as a cake later on.

PREP 20 mins COOK 1 hr 30 mins 9

- 250g rhubarb, cut into 2-3cm lengths
- 275g golden caster sugar
- 1 tsp vanilla bean paste
- 250g vegan margarine, plus extra for greasing
- 2 tbsp ground flaxseed
- 150g soya custard, plus extra to serve (optional)
- 250g self-raising flour
- 1 tsp baking powder
- 1 tsp vanilla extract
- 130g unsweetened apple sauce
- icing sugar, to serve (optional)

1 Heat oven to 200C/180C fan/gas 6. Mix the rhubarb, 25g of the caster sugar and the vanilla paste together in a roasting tin. Bake for 15 mins. Pour away any liquid and leave the rhubarb to cool.

2 Reduce the oven to 170C/150C fan/gas 3½. Grease and line a 25 x 20cm cake tin. Mix the flaxseed with 6 tbsp water in a bowl and leave for 5 mins. Beat the margarine, 100g of the custard, the flour, baking powder, vanilla extract and remaining sugar in a bowl until fluffy, then add the apple sauce and the flaxseed mixture.

3 Put a third of the mixture in the tin and top with a third of the rhubarb. Repeat twice more, then dot teaspoons of the remaining custard on top. Bake for 45 mins, cover with foil and bake for another 30 mins or until golden. Serve warm with soya custard or allow to cool completely, then sprinkle with icing sugar and enjoy as a cake. Eat the same day.

GOOD TO KNOW: Vegan
PER SERVING kcal 274, fat 15g, saturates 3g, carbs 34g, sugars 21g, fibre 2g, protein 2g, salt 0.3g

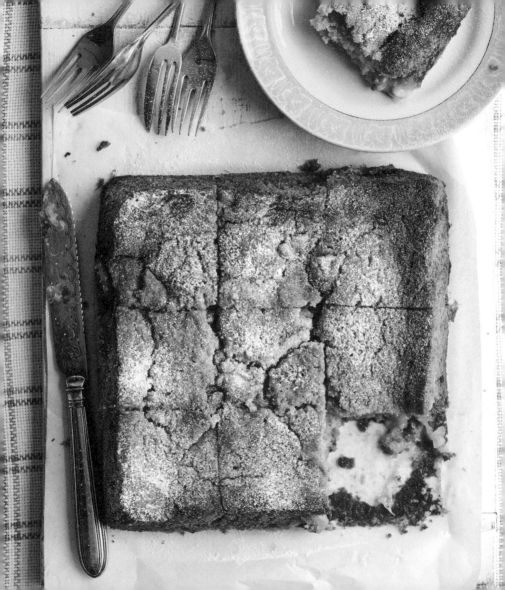

Coconut Nice

· ·

An easy-to-make coconut dough that allows you to whip up a big batch of biscuits for a special occasion.

PREP 30 mins COOK 40 mins (for all the batches)   MAKES around 30

FOR THE BISCUITS
- 1 tbsp linseeds
- 400g plain flour, plus extra for dusting
- 200g coconut oil
- 50g desiccated coconut
- 280g golden caster sugar

FOR THE TOPPING
- 4 tbsp coconut cream
- 200-225g icing sugar
- 50g desiccated coconut

1 Heat oven to 180C/160C fan/gas 4. Soak the linseeds in a bowl with 3 tbsp water for 5-10 mins. Rub the flour and coconut oil together in another bowl until it looks like fresh breadcrumbs. Stir in the desiccated coconut.

2 Blitz the linseeds, their soaking water and the sugar in a food processor until frothy. Pour onto the flour and knead to form a firm dough. Add more water if it feels too dry.

3 Roll out the dough on a floured surface, cut into around 30 rectangles and place on baking sheets lined with baking parchment, leaving a 2-3cm space between each one. Bake in batches for 10-12 mins or until pale golden. Leave to cool.

4 For the topping, mix the coconut cream with enough icing sugar to make a thick paste. Use the paste to stick on the desiccated coconut and to pipe the word 'NICE' on each biscuit, then leave to set.

· ·
GOOD TO KNOW: Vegan
PER SERVING kcal 174, fat 9g, saturates 8g, carbs 20g, sugars 10g, fibre 1g, protein 2g, salt 0g

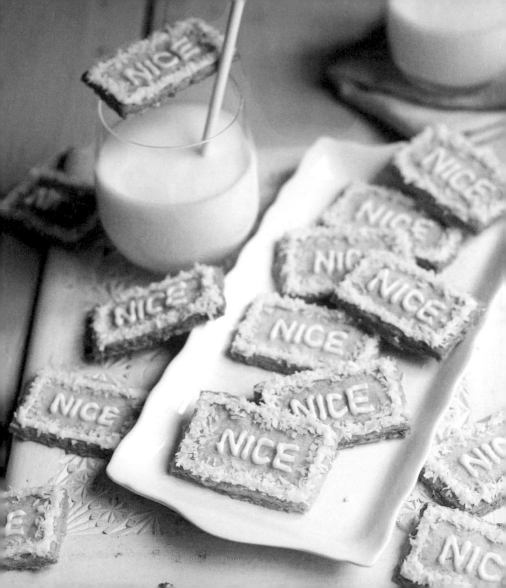

Made-over millionaire's bars

· ·

Just as sticky and moreish as the original millionaire's shortbread, without the dairy.

🕐 PREP 30 mins plus chilling COOK 5 mins   🕐 MAKES 16

FOR THE BASE
- 150g cashew nuts
- 50g rolled oats
- 4 Medjool dates, pitted
- 50g coconut oil, melted

FOR THE FILLING
- 350g pitted Medjool dates
- 125ml unsweetened almond milk
- 25ml maple syrup
- 150g coconut oil
- 1 tsp vanilla extract

FOR THE TOPPING
- 150g coconut oil
- 5 tbsp cocoa powder
- 2 tsp maple syrup

1 Grease and line a 20 x 20cm tin. Blitz the cashews and oats in a food processer until finely chopped. Add the dates and coconut oil, and blitz again. Tip into the tin and press down with the back of a spoon, then chill to firm up.

2 For the filling, put the dates, almond milk, maple syrup and coconut oil in a saucepan with a pinch of salt and bring to a simmer. Boil for 2-3 mins until the dates are soft, then tip into the blender with the vanilla extract and blitz until smooth. Spread over the base and chill.

3 For the topping, gently melt the coconut oil in a saucepan. Remove from the heat and whisk in the cocoa and maple syrup. Cool for 10 mins, pour into the tin and refrigerate for 3 hrs or until set, then cut into squares. Will keep chilled for up to 1 week.

· ·
GOOD TO KNOW: Vegan
PER SERVING kcal 373, fat 28g, saturates 20g, carbs 25g, sugars 20g, fibre 3g, protein 4g, salt 0g

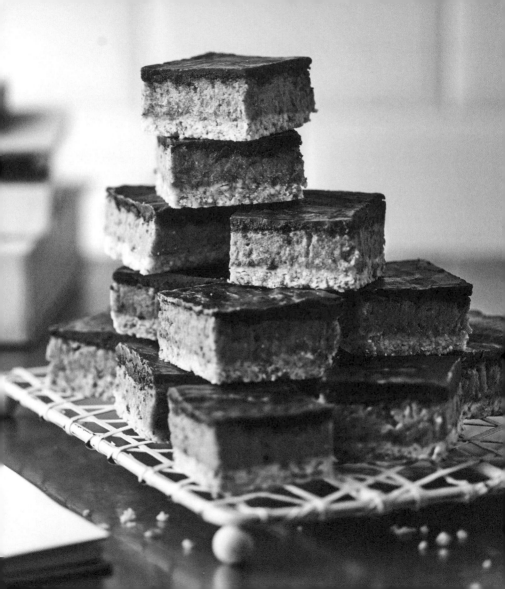

Vegan cherry & almond brownies

An indulgent chocolate-rich treat.

⏱ PREP 20 mins COOK 50 mins ◷ MAKES 12

- 80g vegan margarine, plus extra for greasing
- 2 tbsp ground flaxseed
- 120g vegan dark chocolate
- ½ tsp coffee granules
- 125g self-raising flour
- 70g ground almonds
- 50g cocoa powder
- ¼ tsp baking powder
- 250g golden caster sugar
- 1½ tsp vanilla extract
- 70g glacé cherry (rinsed and halved)

1 Heat oven to 170C/150C fan/gas 3½. Grease and line a 20cm square tin with baking parchment. Combine the flaxseed with 6 tbsp water and set aside for at least 5 mins.

2 In a saucepan, melt the chocolate, coffee and margarine with 60ml water on a low heat. Allow to cool slightly.

3 Put the flour, almonds, cocoa, baking powder and ¼ tsp salt in a bowl and stir to remove any lumps. Using a hand whisk, mix the sugar into the melted chocolate mixture, and beat well until smooth and glossy, ensuring all the sugar is well dissolved. Stir in the flaxseed mixture and vanilla extract, the cherries and then the flour mixture. It will now be very thick. Stir until combined and spoon into the prepared tin. Bake for 35-45 mins until a skewer inserted in the middle comes out clean with moist crumbs. Allow to cool in the tin completely, then cut into squares. Store in an airtight container and eat within 3 days.

GOOD TO KNOW: Vegan
PER SERVING kcal 296, fat 15g, saturates 5g, carbs 36g, sugars 27g, fibre 3g, protein 4g, salt 0.2g

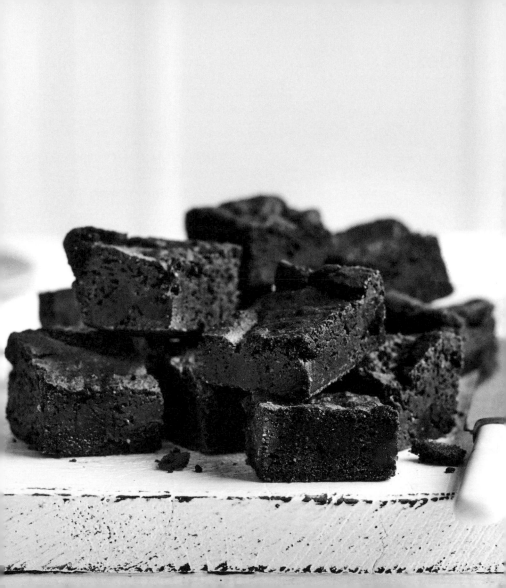

Index

almond
  cranberry & almond clusters 16–17
  Moroccan spiced cauliflower & almond soup 70–1
  rye bread with almond butter & pink grapefruit segments 12–13
  vegan cherry & almond brownies 208–9
apple
  apple croutons 64–5
  cinnamon cashew spread with apple slices 82–3
  green rice with beetroot & apple salsa 114–15
  nutty cinnamon & apple granola 14–15
aubergine
  dukkah-crusted aubergine steaks 122–3
  spiced aubergine bake 144–5
  spicy harissa, aubergine & chickpea soup 62–3
avocado
  avocado panzanella 116–17
  avocado with tamari & ginger dressing 78–9
  California quinoa & avocado salad 108–9
  chocolate avocado cake 198–9
  wholewheat spaghetti & avocado sauce 126–7

banana
  chocolate banana ice cream 184–5
  instant berry banana slush 190–1
  vegan banana & peanut butter cupcakes 200–1
bean(s)
  bean & barley soup 72–3
  Jerk sweet potato & black bean curry 130–1
  kidney bean curry 124–5
  no-cook festival burrito 110–11
  smoky beans on toast 52–3
  summer carrot, tarragon & white bean soup 60–1
  veggie chilli 138–9
beetroot, apple salsa & green rice 114–15
beignets, sweetcorn 58–9
berries
  instant berry banana slush 190–1
  see also specific berries
Bircher, orange & blueberry 26–7
biriyani & carrot salad 142–3
biscuits, coconut Nice 204–5
blueberry
  blueberry & coconut frozen 'cheesecake' bars 188–9
  blueberry chia jam 48–9
  orange & blueberry Bircher 26–7
bread
  flowerpot 162–3
  Indian bread with courgettes & coriander 160–1
  rainbow rolls 168–9
  rye 12–13, 106–7, 166–7
  seeded flatbreads 164–5
  see also croutons; toast
broccoli

  roasted cauli-broc bowl 102–3
  see also Tenderstem broccoli
brownies, vegan cherry & almond 208–9
bulghar salad, crunchy 100–1
burgers, falafel 150–1
burritos, no-cook festival 110–11
butternut squash
  butternut soup with crispy sage & apple croutons 64–5
  green masala butternut squash curry 152–3

cakes
  chocolate avocado cake 198–9
  vegan banana & peanut butter cupcakes 200–1
  see also brownies
cardamom & peach quinoa porridge 10–11
carrot
  carrot & cumin houmous with swirled harissa 84–5
  crushed pea & mint dip with carrot sticks 86–7
  summer carrot, tarragon & white bean soup 60–1
  vegetable vegan biriyani with carrot salad 142–3
cashew cinnamon spread with apple slices 82–3
cauliflower
  Moroccan spiced cauliflower & almond soup 70–1
  roasted cauli-broc bowl 102–3
chai coconut & mango creams 182–3
chard, sweet potato & peanut

stew 140–1
'cheesecake' bars, blueberry & coconut frozen 188–9
cherry
cherries in rosé wine & vanilla syrup 174–5
vegan cherry & almond brownies 208–9
chia
blueberry chia jam 48–9
raspberry ripple chia pudding 22–3
chickpea
bean & barley soup 72–3
carrot & cumin houmous with swirled harissa 84–5
crispy sweet potatoes with chickpeas & tahini yogurt 118–19
falafel burgers 150–1
kadala curry 158–9
keep it green sandwich 106–7
smoky beans on toast 52–3
spicy harissa, aubergine & chickpea soup 62–3
spicy roast chickpeas 80–1
chilli, veggie 138–9
chocolate
choc-orange energy boosters 98–9
chocolate avocado cake 198–9
chocolate banana ice cream 184–5
homemade cocoa pops 20–1
made-over millionaire's bars 206–7
vegan cherry & almond brownies 208–9
cinnamon
cinnamon cashew spread with apple slices 82–3
nutty cinnamon & apple granola 14–15

clementine & honey couscous 30–1
cocoa pops, homemade 20–1
coconut
blueberry & coconut frozen 'cheesecake' bars 188–9
chai coconut & mango creams 182–3
coconut Nice 204–5
key lime & coconut pie 196–7
mango, lime & coconut sundaes 172–3
compote
red berry fruit 180–1
summer fruit 32–3
cookies, oaty hazelnut 194–5
courgette & coriander Indian bread 160–1
couscous
clementine & honey couscous 30–1
dukkah-crusted aubergine steaks 122–3
cranberry & almond clusters 16–17
creams, chai coconut & mango 182–3
croutons
apple 64–5
za'atar 90–1
cucumber raita 128–9
cupcakes, vegan banana & peanut butter 200–1
curry
green masala butternut squash 152–3
Jerk sweet potato & black bean 130–1
kadala 158–9
kidney bean 124–5
spiced okra 134
vegetable vegan biriyani 142–3
custard & rhubarb vegan bake 202–3

dips, crushed pea & mint 86–7
dressings 50, 74, 108, 112
tamari & ginger 78–9
dukkah-crusted aubergine steaks 122–3

energy boosters, choc-orange 98–9

falafel burgers 150–1
filo pastry
spiced pea & potato rolls 94–5
spinach & sweet potato samosa 92–3
flapjacks, feelgood 192–3
flatbread, seeded 164–5
freekeh, spicy vegetable pilau with cucumber raita 128–9
fries, sweet potato 88–9
frosting, choc avocado 198–9

garlic yogurt 50–1
ginger
cheat's pineapple, Thai basil & ginger sorbet 186–7
tamari & ginger dressing 78–9
granola, nutty cinnamon & apple 14–15
grapefruit, rye bread with almond butter & pink grapefruit segments 12–13

harissa
carrot & cumin houmous with swirled harissa 84–5
spicy harissa, aubergine & chickpea soup 62–3
hazelnut oaty cookies 194–5
honey & clementine couscous 30–1
hotpot, Vietnamese veggie 132–3

houmous, carrot & cumin
    houmous with swirled harissa
    84–5

ice cream, choc banana 184–5
icing, peanut butter 200–1
immune boosting smoothie 34–5

jam, blueberry chia 48–9
Jerk sweet potato & black bean
    curry 130–1

kadala curry 158–9
key lime & coconut pie 196–7
kumquat radish salad with
    spice–crusted tofu 112–13

lemon sorbet 176–7
lentil(s)
    lentil ragu with coriander
      136–7
    veggie tahini lentils 120–1
lime
    key lime & coconut pie 196–7
    mango, lime & coconut
      sundaes 172–3

manakeesh 50–1
mango
    chai coconut & mango
      creams 182–3
    mango, lime & coconut
      sundaes 172–3
matcha breakfast bowl 24–5
millionaire's bars, made-over
    206–7
mint
    crushed pea & mint dip with
      carrot sticks 86–7
    minty pineapple smoothies
      42–3
muffins, breakfast 29–30
mushroom & tomato vegan
    pancakes 56–7

noodles
    Japanese tofu noodle bowl
      68–9
    veggie wholewheat pot
      noodle 74–5
    yaki udon 156–7
nutty cinnamon & apple
    granola 14–15

oaty hazelnut cookies 194–5
okra curry, spiced 134
olive, black olive salsa verde
    154–5
orange
    choc-orange energy boosters
      98–9
    orange & blueberry Bircher
      26–7

pancakes
    protein pancake stack 48–9
    tofu brekkie pancakes 54–5
    vegan tomato & mushroom
      pancakes 56–7
panzanella, avocado 116–17
pasta, wholewheat spaghetti &
    avocado sauce 126–7
pea
    crushed pea & mint dip with
      carrot sticks 86–7
    spiced pea & potato rolls 94–5
peach & cardamom quinoa
    porridge 10–11
peanut
    chard, sweet potato & peanut
      stew 140–1
    vegan banana & peanut
      butter cupcakes 200–1
pear, sticky toffee pear pudding
    178–9
pearl barley
    barley & broccoli risotto with
      lemon & basil 148–9
    bean & barley soup 72–3

pie, key lime & coconut 196–7
pineapple
    cheat's pineapple, Thai basil &
      ginger sorbet 186–7
    minty pineapple smoothies
      42–3
porridge
    cardamom & peach quinoa
      10–11
    three-grain 18–19
potato & pea spiced rolls 94–5
puff pastry, slow-roast tomato
    tatin 146–7
pumpkin soup, Thai 76–7

quinoa
    California quinoa & avocado
      salad 108–9
    cardamom & peach quinoa
      porridge 10–11
    protein pancake stack 48–9
    roasted cauli-broc bowl
      102–3

radish kumquat salad with
    spice–crusted tofu 112–13
ragu, lentil ragu with coriander
    136–7
raita, cucumber 128–9
raspberry
    raspberry purée 22–3
    raspberry ripple chia pudding
      22–3
    summer fruit compote 32–3
rhubarb & custard vegan bake
    202–3
rice
    green rice with beetroot &
      apple salsa 114–15
    vegetable vegan biriyani with
      carrot salad 142–3
rose & strawberry sorbet 170–1
rye bread 106–7, 166–7
    rye bread with almond butter

& pink grapefruit segments 12–13

sage, crispy 64–5
salads 50–1
  avocado panzanella 116–17
  California quinoa & avocado 108–9
  crunchy bulghar 100–1
  spice–crusted tofu with kumquat radish 112–13
  vegetable vegan biriyani with carrot 142–3
salsa 58–9
  beetroot & apple 114–15
salsa verde, black olive 154–5
samosa, spinach & sweet potato 92–3
sandwich, keep it green 106–7
seeded flatbreads 164–5
sesame stir-fry wrap 104–5
slush, instant berry banana 190–1
smoky beans on toast 52–3
smoothie bowls
  green rainbow 46
  tropical 44–5
smoothies
  clean green 36–7
  immune boosting 34–5
  minty pineapple 42–3
  sunshine 40–1
  winter warmer 38–9
sorbet
  cheat's pineapple, Thai basil & ginger 186–7
  lemon 176–7
  strawberry & rose 170–1
soup
  bean & barley 72–3
  butternut 64–5
  Indian winter 66–7
  Moroccan spiced cauliflower & almond 70–1

spicy harissa, aubergine & chickpea 62–3
summer carrot, tarragon & white bean 60–1
Thai pumpkin 76–7
spaghetti, wholewheat
spaghetti
  & avocado sauce 126–7
spinach & sweet potato samosa 92–3
spread, cinnamon cashew 82–3
stew, chard, sweet potato & peanut 140–1
sticky toffee pear pudding 178–9
stir-fry wrap, sesame 104–5
strawberry & rose sorbet 170–1
sundae, mango, lime & coconut 172–3
sweet potato
  chard, sweet potato & peanut stew 140–1
  crispy sweet potatoes with chickpeas & tahini yogurt 118–19
  Jerk sweet potato & black bean curry 130–1
  spinach & sweet potato samosa 92–3
  sweet potato fries 88–9
sweetcorn
  sweetcorn beignets 58–9
  yakitori corn pops 96–7
syrup, vanilla 174–5

tahini
  tahini yogurt 118–19
  veggie tahini lentils 120–1
tamari & ginger dressing 78–9
Tenderstem broccoli, barley & broccoli risotto with lemon & basil 148–9
toast, smoky beans on 52–3
toffee pear pudding, sticky 178–9

tofu
  Japanese tofu noodle bowl 68–9
  no-cook festival burrito 110–11
  spice–crusted tofu with kumquat radish salad 112–13
  tofu brekkie pancakes 54–5
  tofu escalope with black olive salsa verde 154–5
tomato
  slow-roast tomato tatin 146–7
  vegan tomato & mushroom pancakes 56–7
tropical smoothie bowl 44–5

vanilla syrup 174–5

wraps
  no-cook festival burrito 110–11
  sesame stir-fry 104–5

yaki udon 156–7
yakitori corn pops 96–7
yogurt
  cucumber raita 128–9
  garlic yogurt 50–1
  tahini yogurt 118–19

za'atar croutons 90–1